No Saints around Here

ALSO BY SUSAN ALLEN TOTH

Blooming: A Small-Town Girlhood

Ivy Days: Making My Way Out East

*How to Prepare for Your High-School Reunion
and Other Midlife Musings*

A House of One's Own (with James Stageberg)

My Love Affair with England

England As You Like It

England for All Seasons

Leaning into the Wind: A Memoir of Midwest Weather

NO SAINTS
AROUND HERE

A Caregiver's Days

Susan Allen Toth

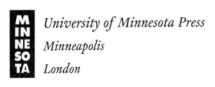

University of Minnesota Press
Minneapolis
London

Published by the University of Minnesota Press
111 Third Avenue South, Suite 290
Minneapolis, MN 55401-2520
http://www.upress.umn.edu

Library of Congress Cataloging-in-Publication Data
Toth, Susan Allen.
No saints around here : a caregiver's days / Susan Allen Toth.
ISBN 978-0-8166-9286-6 (pb : alk. paper)
1. Caregivers. I. Title. PS3620.O887N6 2014
813'.6—dc23
2013034893

Printed in the United States of America on acid-free paper

The University of Minnesota is an equal-opportunity educator and employer.

20 19 18 17 16 15 14   10 9 8 7 6 5 4 3 2 1

For James: then, now, and always

CONTENTS

PREFACE

Caregivers do not forget.

My friend Barb and I were looking together at a realtor's glossy brochure. It was filled with pictures of the house where my husband James and I had lived for twenty-five years. Two years after his death, I had finally acknowledged it was too big and expensive for me. For months I had worked feverishly to dismantle the stuff of our life together.

Grab bars, wheelchair, walker, and hospital bed had long since vanished. As I prepared for sale, I needed to strip to the floorboards and a few pieces of furniture. Out went a chipped enameled stockpot James used for his signature fish soup. A young architect, dear to us both, took James's drawing board. I tossed out the oversize cup James liked to use for coffee. A bedside table he had designed, a wobbly reading lamp we had never replaced, travel posters, a whimsical painted wooden cat with a curly tail that made us smile—everything held a memory. I could dispose of the possessions but not the memories.

"I like those chairs," Barb said, pointing to a picture of two cushy, sagging, lemon-yellow blocks of foam in our upstairs bedroom.

"Yes," I agreed, "so did we. They were so comfy. We both liked to sit there and read." A memory hit. "Remember my telling you about the stupidest thing I ever did when James was starting to have trouble with stairs?"

Barb nodded. "Was that the time when he had a really hard time getting out of a deep chair and then once he was up, he panicked and couldn't move? Is that the chair?" She remembered my story, how eventually I had to call a next-door neighbor to help wrangle James into his lightweight wheelchair and then down two dangerous flights of stairs to his hospital bed in a lower room. Of course I should have called the fire department for a "lift assist." (See "The Last Christmas.")

"I can't believe I did that," I said. "He could have easily fallen out of his wheelchair on the stairs, and that would have been the end. I took such a chance. I was panicked too. I just didn't think straight."

"I get it," Barb said. "I took chances too. Shall I tell you about the dumbest thing I did with Jack?" Her husband had died six years ago. For half an hour, plunged back into what suddenly seemed like a very recent past, we shared stories.

Of course Barb understood. I first met her after Jack's death. Both men had struggled with Parkinson's and eventual related dementia. Barb had cared for Jack at home. When James's neurologist realized I insisted on trying that too, she put me in touch with Barb. I didn't know what to expect. I was twenty years older than Barb, retired from academia, and too occupied with caregiving to continue writing. She was a successful administrator in midcareer, I knew little else about her, and I was not sure how she could help me.

On the sunny July afternoon when I saw Barb walking briskly across the parking lot to my table at an outdoor café, I was even less sure. Tall and slender, she was elegantly dressed in a tailored suit, her hair curled impeccably into a softened helmet, and she carried an official-looking briefcase. I was wearing my usual outfit of well-washed jeans, long-sleeve wild-colored T-shirt, and dangly earrings. My hair felt straggly, and I kept ruffling my fingers through it.

Then Barb dropped her briefcase, slid onto the opposite chair, and reached out her hand. I took it. She looked into my eyes, and as I began to talk, haltingly at first, telling her how long James had been ill, how I wasn't sure what would happen next, how I didn't see how to manage, her eyes filled with tears. "I know," she said over and over. "I know."

We soon became close friends. I grew to depend on an hour's visit with her almost weekly at a coffee shop we could both reach quickly—for different reasons, both of us had almost no spare time—and I could tell her anything. "You can do this," she would say over and over. "You will know when you can't."

My friendship with Barb, and eventually a handful of other caregivers, introduced me into what I now know is an ever-expanding club without borders. In America we number in the millions—current caregiver statistics hover above 46 million and are increasing—of men and women who, meeting in person or in chat rooms or in sponsored groups, almost always instantly understand each other.

Our specific caregiving stories are all different. One of my new friends, suggested by someone who knew us both, had watched early Alzheimer's attack her brilliant, kind husband and had cared for him over the years of his slow decline. Eventually he could not talk or see, and Alice was not even sure he could hear. She was no longer able to lift or move him. When I met her, Alice was driving forty miles round-trip almost every day to visit the only nursing home that would admit him. I never met her husband, but I went to his funeral a few years later. I understood.

For some, caregiving is relatively brief. It may last a few weeks, perhaps months, a year. Those caregivers may—or may not—know when the end may come. They may be able to plan how to expend their energies, and they may—or may not—be able to afford help for a relatively short time.

Others face caring for someone for an indeterminate period that can stretch for so many years that all hope for any independent future seems impossible. Money for help runs out. Another floating statistic claims that almost half of caregivers die before the person for whom the caregiver literally sacrificed his or her life.

James and I were lucky. After he was first diagnosed with Parkinson's, we were able to continue with a gradually changing but still satisfying life for several years. During the last three years, including nine months in hospice care at home, his life and mine constricted. The walls inexorably closed in. But I was able to hire some help when I could no longer cope alone. With help, I was able to keep going. Four days before he died, even assisted by a sturdy aide, I could no longer turn him in bed. I knew that day I was soon facing what he and I had always dreaded: an institution. Then James suddenly developed pneumonia, and within twenty-four hours, he was gone. He died at home. He was surrounded by love. That is why I say we were lucky.

Caregivers carry different burdens. Some are helping an elderly mother, father, or other aging relative through a final passage. Some have to watch their parents or siblings die far too young. Others—a deep and terrible fear that most parents cannot even bear to acknowledge as a possibility—have to watch their children die. Many of us have partners or spouses, and as we see them begin to leave us, we know that the intricately woven fabric of our lives is disintegrating. We look ahead into a void.

Despite the varying details of our specific lives, caregivers all know about grief, despair, exhaustion, frustration, unexpected crises, surprising sources of support, and the relief of sharing our stories. We can talk honestly together about our mistakes, anger, embarrassment, and guilt, stories no one else could hear and honestly respond, "Oh, of course. That happened to me too. Lots of times." We can even laugh, edgily but openly, about moments of black humor that to an outsider might sound heartless.

We know we are not heartless. We don't need to talk much about love. Love defines itself in many ways, but it was a bedrock on which we all—sometimes shakily—stood. After the person we loved died, we still keep that love for balance. A few sentences echo among us: "I loved her so much." "He told me I was his angel." "She smiled whenever I came into the room." "I was the only one he trusted." "When she could no longer speak, she would reach out to touch my cheek." "I miss him so much."

"So much." I think that simple phrase could easily be the motto emblazoned on a caregiver's shield. Love, pain, courage, endurance, loss. So much, so much.

Hearing others' stories helped me continue. In the following pages, I tell some of my own. After my introduction, they appear in chronological order, as I wrote them during James's last eighteen months. How they began, and how, in slightly different form, some led a brief and almost invisible life as a pseudonymous blog, forms part of my narrative too.

Besieged by thoughts and feelings not always easy to express, a caregiver can often feel quite alone. All caregivers have a lot to say, and we all need someone to hear us. This memoir is one way of starting a conversation.

INTRODUCTION

Endings and Beginnings

Sometime after midnight, I finally fell into an exhausted, drugged, but uneasy sleep. When Jeanne, my aide that night, tapped me lightly on the shoulder at 2:00 a.m., I was instantly awake. I knew before she spoke.

"Susan," she said gently, "he's gone."

In one moment, I was out of bed and down the stairs. I don't remember exactly what I felt in those seconds—mostly, I think, numb, as if I had been stunned by a hammer.

In the lower bedroom, my husband James, gray, gaunt, and motionless, lay on his hospital bed. Even though Parkinson's had begun its slow destructive work almost fourteen years before, I had never thought James—who, at eighty-five, had still managed to keep a gleam in his eye—seemed shockingly old. Now he did.

He looked much as I had left him two hours before, his mouth wide open, jaw dropped, as though he were fighting to breathe. But he was not breathing anymore. He was motionless. When I reached to touch his face, it was still hot with fever.

He was gone. I had not been there. No matter that Mary, our hospice nurse, had told me a few hours earlier, when she arrived with morphine to ease James's breathing, "This could go on for days. It could go on for a week." No matter that I knew if I had to last for days I would need some sleep. I was not there when he died.

I had been sure I would be there.

Several years earlier, on a freezing winter afternoon just before Christmas, when James could still drive downtown to his architectural office, he slipped and fell on an icy sidewalk. I had long ago stuck a little card into his wallet with a warning that James was taking Coumadin, a blood thinner, as well as our doctor's name and phone number.

When I picked up the phone that afternoon, Eben, our doctor and old friend, told me quickly what had happened. "James is on the way to Abbott Northwestern. He fell on the sidewalk outside his office. Someone called 911. He regained consciousness before the ambulance arrived. You'll want to go to the emergency room right away."

As I raced to the hospital, trying to fight off visions of broken bones, blood clots, and brain hemorrhages, I concentrated on saying to myself, "Red light. Stop. Green light. Go. Left lane. Slow down. Don't hit anyone." I also thought, "I should have known this would happen."

I was in the emergency room twenty minutes later. As I hurried into James's cubicle, a doctor, just leaving, said someone would come in a few minutes to take James for an MRI. James gave me a dazed, uncertain smile. After kissing him—I didn't dare do much more than stroke his face gently—I grabbed a chair and pulled it up to his bedside. "I knew you'd be here," he said. "I told them, 'Susan will be here.'"

At that moment, lying on the emergency room table, James did not know what day it was, or what month, or what had happened. He could not tell me. When he had been loaded into the ambulance, he would not have been able to ask someone to call me. But I was struck that even in his blurred, half-conscious state, James could still say with such assurance, "Susan will be here." Because he needed me, he knew I would come.

Astonishingly, James had only suffered a concussion and bruises. Hours later, we were home.

But I never forgot his weak yet absolutely confident voice: "I told them, 'Susan will be here.'" I could not know then how his faith would sustain me in the years ahead.

On the morning before he died, when I returned from the grocery store, I noticed James looked warm. After Martha, my main daily aide, took his temperature, I was shaken. "He almost never runs a fever," I said to her. "Not for months." The thermometer registered 100°F; an hour later, 100.5°F. I called Mary. She said she would come as soon as she could.

At breakfast, I had spoon-fed James some tapioca pudding. He had choked and coughed for a few moments. Even now, I find myself wondering if I had fed him too much, too fast.

At any time, advanced Parkinson's patients with dementia can die of many causes: falls, broken hips, concussion; weakness from lack of absorbing nutrients; inability to swallow, hence choking; swallowing wrong—too much tapioca on the spoon?—hence infection in the lungs, then pneumonia.

Already James had been in a hospital-based hospice program for nine months—at least six months longer, I'd been told, than the average hospice patient. In February, Mary said the end wasn't far. In June, I wondered if he would hang on until August. No one could answer me.

The Middle

I also did not know how much longer I could continue my caregiving at home. I wanted with my whole heart to do this. I could not imagine James anywhere but in the home he had designed and loved. He had lived there more than thirty years.

I knew I couldn't promise him that. I could only try. For his last three years, James needed someone with him all the time. One stumble, one missed stair could mean disaster. Then, no more stairs. A walker, almost useless in his confined space. Someone's steady hand on his elbow. A heavy-duty transfer belt with handles for grabbing and guidance. Complicated gymnastics to the commode or shower. More assistance needed. Then even more.

Although I used this overworked phrase myself, I came to hate the flipness of "24/7." Those snap-tight numbers cannot convey the unrelenting intensity and stress of caregiving. In James's case, I didn't feel that immediately. After he had been diagnosed, we continued for almost seven years to lead fairly normal lives—modified a little at first, then more, then increasingly restricted. "More" is a word I learned to use often, balancing it with "less": less mobility, less activity, less awareness, less communication. More adjustments. More changes. More help. Always less—and always more.

I never wanted to look very far down our road. I knew where it would end, but not the twists, dizzying curves, and detours it would take. Instead of trying to peer through an opaque and terrifying mist, I mostly kept my eyes on my feet: one step forward, another step. Step, step, pause. Step, step, keep going.

We did not talk very much about what lay ahead. A very few times during his long bout with Parkinson's, feeling frightened, James asked me, "What is going to happen?" He did not mention the word "dying" until very close to the end.

I could honestly tell him I didn't know. "Well," I'd say, "you have Parkinson's. Parkinson's doesn't get better. You are fifteen years older than I am. Odds are that you will reach the farther shore before I do. But nobody knows. I could be hit by a bus tomorrow." (He grimaced.) "I could," I insisted. "Life is always uncertain. I don't know what is going to happen. So we just keep going." He nodded, I hugged him, and we marched on.

Until James could no longer walk, even with assistance, we actually did march. Always an active man, he often felt restless. He could no longer jog or bike, but for a long while he could walk, with gradually increasing difficulty. Like many Parkinson's patients' experience, at times his muscles would suddenly stop working. He needed a signal, a rhythm, that would jolt his beleaguered brain into sending the right message to his legs.

So I would start to sing. In a few moments, gallant and unwilling to give up, he would join me. Neither of us had a very good voice. (James's was worse.) I could, however, sing quite loudly. As I held tightly to his transfer belt and he clutched his cane, we marched around his room, up the stairs—until he could no longer climb stairs—and in circles around our living room and kitchen.

Although James was born in 1925 and I in 1940, we shared much of the same popular music. At my high school formals, a live band often played Glenn Miller, and our disc jockey dances always closed with "Stardust." When my daughter Jenny was a teenager in the 1980s, she was appalled to learn that I had never moved much further than Frank Sinatra, Doris Day, Elvis Presley, and the Beatles. So James and I could sing some of the same songs.

To keep him moving, our favorites were "There's a Long, Long Trail A-winding," "Don't Fence Me In," and "Side by Side," with lilting melodies and emphatic rhythms. For James, they also held memories that stretched back to World War II. As he grew weaker, the lyrics began to seem achingly poignant to me, but I don't think James noticed. He was concentrating too hard on moving his feet.

We kept marching until he could not walk at all.

Since I understood Parkinson's, though progressive and incurable, varied with everyone, I tried to pretend that James would never have to suffer its worst effects. My denial was partly based on James's spirit. James battled fiercely to keep his body and mind moving and in balance. An ebullient man, he wanted to continue to enjoy life as much as he could. After James's death, a friend of his told me, "I remember when James was still able to go out to lunch. I commiserated with him one day about his Parkinson's and told him how much I admired his attitude. And he replied,

'Well, I can't do anything about having Parkinson's, but I don't have to get depressed about it.'"

Of course James did get depressed. So did I. Loving, resilient, and funny, but fully human, he wasn't a saint, and I certainly wasn't either. I don't like to remember now—but I can't always help myself—the times I snapped at him, lost my temper, and (more than once) literally tore at my hair in frustration. "Oh, James, I told you not to walk down those steps without calling me!" "*Can't* you let me finish my meal, just this once?" "You don't like this movie? Well, what in the world can I find for you to do now? I've run out of ideas!" I can hear my angry voice, and I can also hear, even more painfully, his soft, hurt answer, like a child's, "Please don't scold me, Susan." That always made me instantly subside into shame.

In spite of his own occasional irritation and depression, James would always somehow fight his way back. He had a remarkable ability to focus on the pleasures he could still enjoy. Even when dementia began to disorient him, he did not give up. About a week before he died, propped up in his hospital bed, James was mesmerized by a DVD of *Swan Lake*. Although we had seen only a handful of live ballets together, James had loved them. On that afternoon, I marveled as James—his attention span limited, unable to read or even listen to someone reading—concentrated all his waning powers on Margot Fonteyn and Rudolf Nureyev. They floated across the screen, leaping and whirling, immortal in their grace and fluidity.

Until he was past seventy, James delighted, like a teenager with a mischievous smile, in showing how he could jump into the air and click his heels. Not too high, but a definite click. I think of this as quintessential James. Now, lying on his bed, he could no longer turn over or even move from one side to another without help. As Tchaikovsky's compelling melodies poured into the room, I could not watch any more. I had to get up and leave.

When I left the room, Martha stayed. Here I need to state

clearly and emphatically: I had paid part-time help. Long-term caregiving can be very, very expensive. Except for a few hours a week, in-home assistance is not a Medicare benefit. High-quality nursing homes are out of reach of most people. Although I worried about how our retirement account was draining away, month by month, with an almost audible sucking sound, I never had to sell our house or apply for Medicaid. James and I were very fortunate.

Sometimes I browsed among caregiver sites on the Internet, where contributors often posted frantic, despairing cries on community bulletin boards. They were running out of money; they were running out of physical strength. If I had been much older, if I had not been able to take occasional breaks or to hire aides to help (especially at night), I do not know if I would have lasted. Many caregivers don't.

Not every aide was easy to have around. A very, very few were irritating, difficult, or maddening. But all were compassionate and loving to James. They worked hard. At different times, I needed every one of them.

I was also lucky. Both in print and online, scary stories sometimes describe aides who have stolen, lied, behaved very badly, and—not as serious, but also devastating—simply failed to show up for their scheduled shifts. I have seen how focused and attentive they must be, I know they are usually underpaid for work that is physically and emotionally demanding, and so I am not always shocked by these tales.

When my small, comforting circle of other caregivers, past and present, occasionally grumbled or dryly reminisced to me about one or another of their aides, they never reported anything legally actionable. But they all struggled now and then. Living closely together, under trying circumstances, caregiver and aide have to negotiate many daily details about who is in charge, who should do what, and how it should be done. Small annoyances can slowly rise to the surface, and, unless I could rush outdoors for a fast walk, call a sympathetic friend, or retreat into a bedroom and bash a pillow, everything might have coalesced and breached like an unexpectedly explosive whale. A whale? Wild exaggeration? No. Caregivers (like me) do sometimes lose a sense of proportion.

"One day I couldn't stand it any longer," said my friend Dolores, whose husband had died a few months before. "I finally had to tell my main aide, Kathleen, who was really a good person at heart, a cock-and-bull story about a cousin of mine who was going to come to help me, so I wouldn't need her anymore. The thing is," Dolores went on, almost apologetically, "Kathleen talked all the time. I mean, *all* the time, from the moment she entered my door until she left in the afternoon. We had no children, and I had always lived in a quiet house. After a few hours I was going nuts.

"She always wore bright blue uniforms, I think because she had never finished her nursing degree and wanted to appear official. Kathleen had to be right all the time. She questioned every decision I made, and since she had experience in practical nursing, and of course I didn't, I usually gave in. She wanted to discuss every detail of Charlie's care, and she had already decided what she was going to do before she asked. She commented on everything—what time the mailman came, what I was fixing for my lunch, why the dog was sleeping on the sofa. Blah, blah, blah. Even her constant fluty giggles finally got to me. She giggled almost as much as she talked. Finally, at the end of one interminable day, I thought to myself, 'I feel as if I'm being pecked to death by bluebirds.'

"The next day, I started looking for someone else." Dolores looked guilty.

I understood. I also understood how my friend Louise had felt. Although her husband had died many years before, Louise remembered one particular day when, she confessed, she wanted to murder her long-term aide, Carrie. As months of caregiving went on, Louise told me she had found herself relying on Carrie more and more. "She took such good care of John," said Louise, "and so I guess I gradually let her take over more and more. When I went into John's room, she made me feel as if I were interrupting. I think maybe she forgot who was the wife. But on the other hand, she'd also say things like, 'Should I leave you two lovebirds alone for a while?' and smile sweetly. I felt so awkward. How was I supposed to answer that?

"The problem was," Louise continued, "I really needed Carrie. I didn't know how I could ever replace her. John was used to her. I knew she was supporting her divorced daughter, who had recently lost her job. How could I possibly fire her? I felt I was stuck. Then when John went into hospice care at home, Carrie took a great dislike to our visiting nurse, Tilda. Tilda was funny, easy, breezy, and a great breath of fresh air. She listened politely to Carrie's reports, which always went on too long, but then Tilda made her own decisions about John's care. I could see Carrie hated that. I would say something to Tilda, and Carrie would contradict me. She could get quite insistent. Cheerfully and unflappably, Tilda just ignored her.

"So one afternoon after Tilda's weekly visit, when Carrie was quietly fuming, I walked Tilda to her car. I couldn't help myself. I said, 'Someday I'm going to murder that woman.' Tilda stopped, looked straight at me, and smiled. 'Not if I get there first,' she said firmly, and then she turned and opened her car door. I loved Tilda."

Having help was a life-saving privilege, but—not being a saint—I too chafed under the pressures that help necessarily brought. I missed my privacy. When James and I were alone together, I never felt crowded. He was, in fact, the only person in my whole life I never needed to get away from. With an aide in the house, all that changed. I was always on call. I chose to be available—I felt I absolutely had to be available—for consultation, disturbing or encouraging bulletins on daily developments, even just an extra set of hands. I lived with constant interruptions.

My initial experience with an agency was not a happy one. The agency, licensed and reputable, mostly sent us aides who seemed brusque and bored. They did not like what they were doing, and that showed. One day I found Luke, a new arrival, sitting on our outdoor steps, staring at nothing, because he said James had told him he wasn't needed right now. I decided to find my own helpers. Recommendations from friends, and then suggestions from the aides I found, in time provided a team of lifesavers. I started with just one who came only a few hours each week. Gradually I added more hours and then more helpers. I hesitated each time as I did. Not only did I fret about cost, but I knew James would need to adjust to yet another stranger.

Luckily, James accepted these changes with incredible patience and understanding. All I had to do was explain how tired I was and how more help would keep us further from a nursing home. It mattered enormously that James had never been self-conscious about his body. (In fact, when he had been able to move freely, he sometimes wandered blithely straight from his bath into an upstairs room whose large window faced the street. He scoffed as I raced behind him to pull the shades.)

James always blanched when I used the words "nursing home." Once, when I warned him that if he persisted in walking without his cane, he might fall and end up in a nursing home— I was not above such threats—he said, flinching, "I can't imagine a worse fate." Without help, I am sure that day would have arrived long before the end.

Since I had some help, I could take care of myself in ways that would not have been otherwise possible. In James's last few years, as caregiving grew ever more strenuous, our doctor and close friends urged me to take a longer break than my usual day or weekend—a week, maybe even nine or ten days. Occasionally, head pounding and teeth clenched, I drove two hours each way for as little as twenty-four solitary hours, possibly a day or two more, in our wooded Wisconsin retreat, and even in such a short time, I was refreshed. Best of all, I once spent four nights in Seattle, a city I barely knew, with trusted, intimate friends who pulled me out of a threatening depression with stimulating conversation, delicious food and wine, and interesting excursions I didn't have to plan.

Now, one friend told me, I needed more. "Or else," Grace said, "I'm not sure you'll make it. I've been watching you these last months. You're beyond tired, you seem frantic, you're jumpy. I don't want to sound dramatic, but you can't let this awful disease claim two people." At first I thought I couldn't possibly be away from James for very long. A week? Nine days? I thought that over. I thought some more.

Feeling guilty (all that money!), worried (how would James react to my absence?), frightened (did I still know how to travel alone?), I took the boldest step I could imagine. I arranged a solo nine-day trip to London, a very familiar city. Three of my books are memoirs about James's and my travels in the U.K. I knew how to cherish its distractions. Glaringly cognizant that few caregivers could hope for such a break, I felt embarrassed about it. I found myself trying not to mention my trip to many people.

(How I got there is part of the story that follows this introduction. Like everything in a caregiver's life, my departure had its own unexpected drama. I wrote "At the Foot of the Roller Coaster" as I waited in the Minneapolis airport to board my plane.)

Even taking a break is not simple for a caregiver. Recently I found a calendar page I'd printed out for my planning process. I had to consult each of my aides separately, with countless phone calls, e-mails, and emendations. Finally I could write a daily schedule on each calendar square: Wednesday, Sandy 8:00 to 1:00, Trish 1:00 to 6:00 p.m., Amy 6:00 and overnight to 8:00 a.m.; Thursday, Martha 8:00 to 8:00, Jeanne 8:00 and overnight; on and on. I entered notes for emergency backups.

Then I wrote out menu plans; I cooked and bought and froze main dishes and desserts; I rented DVDs and piled up books that

James might enjoy. I made many lists. I bought a cheap calling card and told my aides I would phone twice a day. I explained how they could reach me in any emergency. For each day I would be gone, I left an envelope for James with a loving message and a photo. Since I would be seeing some places he and I knew well, maybe he could remember and picture me there.

A break from caregiving can seem surreal. I walked through the looking glass into London. Once there, dazed by unaccustomed freedom, I walked, rode buses, zoomed here and there on the Underground, walked some more, visited a few museums, and often forgot everything for a few hours in darkened theaters. But what I most vividly remember was lying on a couch. It sat next to a floor-to-ceiling window in my second-floor rented flat on busy Lower Sloane Street. As the red double-decker buses rumbled past, I could look into their top decks. People seated next to the bus windows stared for a moment through mine and then disappeared. All those people riding somewhere, and I didn't have responsibility for any of them. I just lay there, adrift in anonymity, letting the world roll by. I could not remember when I had felt so peaceful.

Coming home from a break is a revelation. When I returned from London, I felt my glasses had been cleaned, foggy residue wiped away, clear vision restored. I dropped my suitcase in the hall and hurried up the stairs to the bedroom. James was seated in his wheelchair. Although it was past his usual bedtime, he had been determined to wait until I arrived. He smiled when he saw me. As I hugged him, he said, "I thought maybe you weren't ever coming home."

"Oh, you know better than that," I said. "You'll never get rid of me. Never."

He smiled again. I was shocked at how thin and frail he looked. I saw how much his illness had really progressed, so slowly over the last few months that I had not fully registered its continued depredations.

My time away had given me a new perspective. Within an hour of arriving home, I knew I needed to make plans to settle James into another room. I could now see that it was too dangerous for him to maneuver the short flight of stairs to the main bathroom. A lower bedroom had an adjacent shower. I would have to clean and refurnish that smaller room and make it comfortable and welcoming for him—very soon.

Late that night, jet-lagged and strung out, I sat at my computer to learn about hospital beds. It was probably time for that too. The jolts didn't end there. Scrolling blearily through Internet pages of information about hospital beds, I understood I had put off talking to an in-home hospice program for far too long. Only a few weeks following my return, after looking at our options and then consulting with our doctor, I made that call.

All these necessary changes would have happened eventually. But now I had the strength to tackle them. I was profoundly grateful for my team of aides, assisted during my absence by two of James's grown children. By taking on his entire care for my time away, they had made it possible for me to continue.

The days, weeks, and months passed, and somehow we all managed. To my infinite relief, James never had to go into the nursing home he dreaded. One morning soon after his death, I drove to a nearby coffee shop to meet my widowed and former caregiver friend Barb. As we startled the coffee drinkers around us with our vigorous, pumping high fives, we both had tears in our eyes. We had done it.

The Beginning: Finding the Words

I did not begin writing about caregiving until eighteen months before James died. I am not sure why I waited that long. Perhaps I was too immersed in trying to keep our lives as rich as possible and would not allow myself the time. More likely, I did not want to confront my conflicting feelings, including terror, sorrow, anger, despair, and a love that made the thought of losing James unimaginable. I have never been able to keep a journal. Although I jotted brief paragraphs and notes onto my computer, they lay there as scattered outbursts.

Finally, out of desperation, I started to write. I had a daughter. I had good friends. I even, thank God, had a wise and understanding therapist. In her office, I could always tell the truth. None of this was enough. As a writer, I instinctively turned to language. If I could give my experience a shape, this might help make it endurable. I needed to seek some sense of control over what was happening to James and to me.

So often I felt helpless. I remember the first moment when I sensed our life together begin to tilt on its axis. Ten years before James died, Eben, doctor and dear friend, took me aside one evening after a supper together. "I don't want you to think I haven't noticed James's tremor," he said. I had barely registered how James's left hand sometimes shook slightly, but I knew instantly what Eben was telling me.

"Parkinson's?" I asked, unbelieving.

"Perhaps," Eben said.

After a small, unexplained stroke at the age of seventy-one a few years before, my vibrant, lighthearted, and lively husband had almost entirely recovered, except for that tremor. He went every day to his architectural office, and he still plunged into his projects with the passion that suffused his entire life. Yes, he tired more easily. His enthusiastic, fluent conversation—he had always told long, complicated, and groaningly hilarious shaggy-dog stories—was sometimes more halting. He did not walk as fast and as confidently as before. In energy and speed, for the first time he no longer outpaced me, fifteen years younger. But Parkinson's?

Eben was right. A few months later James was diagnosed by the neurologist at our regional Parkinson's center. Since I am a lifetime reader, imbued with the certainty that answers often lie in someone's story on the printed page, I began to buy books. Quite frightening books about Parkinson's; often illuminating and very moving memoirs about caring for a parent, a spouse, or a child with a fatal disease; then, as James's illness progressed, devastating memoirs about caring for someone with dementia.

But I was also looking for something more. I wanted a report from the front lines. I wanted details. In all the memoirs I consulted, the writers were looking backward. They shared their stories from a considered distance. No one gave me an unblinkered, running account as caregiving gradually grew from a mild nuisance to a constant worry to an all-consuming way of life.

The little things, not just the big stuff: that is what I wanted to hear.

No one told me how she (or he) felt when she had to brush and floss her husband's teeth.

So one cold winter afternoon, as an aide stayed with James, I fled to a nearby mall, a small, uncrowded place, where an out-of-the-way nook provided a few tables and chairs. There, with my laptop, a sandwich, and a mug of decaf, I turned some notes into my first finished essay. I was thinking of future readers, other caregivers, who had neither the time nor the words to describe and share their own experiences. As I tried to understand what was happening to me, I was also writing for them. I was talking to someone who might not know anything about me yet—but who might someday want to know what my caregiving was like.

I kept writing: short pieces, longer ones, sometimes close together, often not for weeks. For a time, I posted some on a pseudonymous blog. It barely created a ripple on the vast and intricate Web. That didn't matter. I continued to write. I wrote the final dated entry just days after James died. For this book, I added one more: "A Ring among the Ashes."

Soon after James died, I promised myself that I would return to my accumulated pages, neatly printed out in a folder, and re-read them. When I wrote these essays, I filed them and seldom looked back. I thought I would assess what I'd done some weeks after his death.

But I couldn't.

More than a year later, I understood why. For many months I had remained almost as shocked as I was that phantasmagoric night of July 7, when Jeanne woke me and whispered in my ear, "He's gone." I kept moving; I did things; I talked to people. Unbelievably, life went on. I coped. Although grief sometimes washed over me in terrible waves, I almost never wept. "Let it out," urged my sister. So did my therapist. I couldn't. My tears were buried beyond reach.

For a long time I convulsively clung to the sense that James was still with me. (I continue to feel this, though in a quieter, indefinable way, and I hope I always will.) Perhaps that is what explains what happened three nights after he died. That night, the house was completely quiet, and I was deep into a dreamless sleep. Then I woke with a start. I thought I heard a noise. Sitting up with a stab of fear, I saw James standing in the dark at the foot of our bed.

My first thought was one of joy. I leaped out of bed and hugged him tightly. He looked good, not especially young or animated, but not ill or emaciated. He was smiling. "Oh, James, I am so glad to see you," I said, my voice quavering. "I miss you so much. Are you okay?"

Of course I knew James was dead. But I meant, wherever you are, are you all right?

"I'm okay," James said. I wasn't sure I liked the way he said this. He seemed a little hesitant. He wasn't joyful. At the moment—and later, when I recalled this experience—I felt vaguely disappointed and even worried. I suppose I wanted him to say something more comforting than "okay."

Instantly I wanted to reassure him in return. "You know, darling," I said soothingly, snuggling into him, feeling his closeness, "I'm past seventy now. I'll be joining you before too much longer."

"Oh, good!" he said, hugging me tighter. He sounded quite pleased.

Then I felt alarmed. I'd better clarify this. "Not that soon," I said hastily. "No, no, not *that* soon. You'll have to wait a while."

James said nothing. I thought he looked a little sad. We held on to each other for a very brief time. I don't know how long, but it didn't seem long enough.

Then I woke up. I had pushed myself into a half-sitting position, probably from hearing that earlier noise, and James—if he had indeed been there—was gone. Except in later dreams, when I definitely knew I was dreaming, James never returned.

This was an intensity I did not want to relive in my reading—not just yet. A few months after his death, I decided to escape not just our grieving house but also the impending Minnesota winter. So I fled to a rented apartment in La Jolla, California, where I knew almost no one, and I emerged into bewildering but welcome sunshine. I took my essays with me, packed into a cardboard box they filled tidily. I would read them in La Jolla, I told myself.

I didn't. The box sat—looking, in an unsettling way, rather like the cardboard box of James's ashes (see "A Ring among the Ashes")—under a small end table on the living room floor. All was in order. The box fit that space quite snugly. It didn't seem to want to be moved. From time to time, I regarded it with a question mark in my mind. Then I left the box where it was and walked out my door to look at the ocean.

When I returned to Minneapolis in early spring, my numbness had begun to wear off. I was now distracted, distressed, and increasingly unsure about what I was going to do with the rest of my life. Almost immediately after unpacking, I drove to Lakewood Cemetery. In the section where James's ashes lie, all the plaques are alike: small, dignified, metal, with clear but unshowy lettering. I stood in front of his plaque and noticed that his lettering shone so much more brightly than the surrounding markers. After eight months, it was still brand-new. His ashes might have been buried yesterday.

That was when I started to cry. I cried, and I talked aloud. No one was in that part of the cemetery, and I wasn't the least embarrassed. I knew what lay below wasn't James, but I talked to him anyway. This felt like the right place to do it. I had lots to say, some of the same words over and over. Mostly I said, "I miss you so much, James. I just miss you so much. I don't know what to do. I miss you so much. I don't know what to do. I don't know what to do." Later I found a nearby bench. I sat there until I felt ready to drive home.

Now, I thought later that day. Maybe now is the time to open the box. I need to be writing again. James would want this. He always encouraged me, even prodded when I was away from my writing too long. Again I couldn't. So many months later, yet everything was still too raw.

Weeks passed. Although other widows had warned me about the possible seismic effects of anniversaries, I had thought to myself, "No, no. James and I never made a fuss about special dates, except maybe birthdays." I was wrong. I sank into dread for at least a week before and after July 7. The night of July 7 was like reliving a nightmare. Then, after that night, I was better able to face reality. James was gone. I was older. I looked ahead to the looming end of summer and the beginning of fall, and I thought, "It's time." I postponed opening the box for a few more days—I cleaned a closet, I weeded my backyard garden, I roasted vegetables—but finally I sat down and began.

I had always promised myself that if I ever assembled my essays into a full-length manuscript, I would not change anything. I would keep my entries as I had first written them, fraught with the urgency of each particular time, and I would not edit or alter my text.

As I reread, I amended my original determination. First I sliced a few digressions that sounded flat or boring. Then, as I slowly turned the pile of pages, I noticed how often I repeated myself. I allowed some repetitions to stay because they were part of my story.

"I have no time," for instance, is a refrain that occurs again and again. Caregivers are sensitive to time in many ways. Even if we do not know the date, we gradually understand that our remaining time with the person we love is finite. I struggled with this uncertainty, which is reflected in many of my essays, sometimes wanting this long siege—and the continuing deterioration it wreaked—to end. I did not know how much longer I could go on. And then sometimes I would look at James, whom I loved so much, and wonder how I could ever let such thoughts enter my mind.

All my life I have been busy. Temperamentally, like James, I am very active and energetic, and I try to cram too much into each day. I thought I knew what overload felt like, especially since I raised my daughter alone after she was two years old while I was teaching full-time at a local college. A single working mother never has enough time. But a caregiver has even less. In those years alone with Jenny, before I married James, I baked bread. I went to movies. I took Jenny for haircuts, play dates, and short trips. I even wrote books. How did I ever find the time? Did I feel then I was living like a hamster in a cramped cage? I don't think so.

In the essays I reread, I could hear a monotonous undertone, an unsettled or angry or resentful voice muttering, "Time. Time. There is no time." I heard it even in passages where I didn't think I was writing about time. I found myself once jotting in the margin of my manuscript, "Where did the day go? How did I disappear?"

I was startled to discover that I complain with discomfiting frequency about not being able to finish my breakfast tea. I have always enjoyed eating breakfast, and all my life, unless I had stomach flu, I never, ever skipped that critical meal. I relish—I depend on—two large mugs of Earl Grey tea with milk together with my eggs or cereal. Not being able to sip my tea in a leisurely and uninterrupted way became a metaphor for my sense of truncated time.

A missed cup of tea—even repeated missed cups of tea—is a very small loss. Small losses, trivial routines, supposedly harmless comments: these were often the twigs that fueled a blazing fire. Going through my essays, I thought more than once, "I'm complaining about brushing his teeth *again*? Everyone will assume I did nothing but brush James's teeth. Do I ever sound petty! How could that be such a big deal?" Because it was a big deal. I performed many other, more time-consuming, and even more intimate tasks without any sense of grievance. Yet brushing and flossing my beloved husband's teeth—a necessity he uncharacteristically fought right up to the end—was a continued blow to both of us.

Much of this litany of complaints remains intact in the essays that follow. I also left in most of my repeated comments—muttering and moaning—about fatigue. I was always tired. Inexplicably, perhaps because I was determined to exercise most days and because, loving food, I tried to eat well and because—once again—I had help, I remember being sick only once or twice in the last three years of caregiving. But I never felt rested.

Close to the end, I had several dizzy spells. I interpreted them as urgent messages from my body that I simply had to stop. Each time I lay down on the sofa, closed my eyes, and rested until my head was clear again. Since James's death, this has only recurred twice, at times of great weariness and stress, and I now know what to do. I give up; I have no choice.

I fought depression and lack of energy as best I could, and here too, reliving those weeks, months, and years in my entries, I discovered the importance of trivia. Did I actually write about the morale-boosting significance of buying a new pair of jeans? Yes. Or about staring at eBay, too tired to do anything except watch colors and textures scroll down my screen? Yes. Did I call up my daughter in a disbelieving, barely controlled hysteria to tell her I had just painted Wite-Out on a bleeding cut? I did.

I also noted how much I wrote about food. Not long ago, I had supper with an old friend, also a fairly recent widow. When Dolores opened her refrigerator door, she said, "Oh, Susan, can you believe this? It's only me, and I have all these shelves stuffed. I can't even find room to stash your bottle of wine. Isn't this awful?"

"No," I reassured her. "My fridge is just as full. We need to nurture ourselves. That's what all this food represents. You don't want to open that door and find yourself looking at only half a lemon green with mold, a quart of skim milk, and lettuce brown at the edges."

During James's long illness, I spent much of my time trying to nurture him—and myself—with good food. I was not surprised to see my last essay before he died, which even includes a recipe, is called "French Toast." Feeding James was often a frustrating process. On days when he pushed aside his plate and said flatly and firmly, "I just don't like the way this tastes," I could feel another dry, combustible twig drop. And sometimes I struck the match.

His Head Is in the Pansies

What often kept me from going up in flames was unexpected laughter. Humor, slanted or slapstick or ludicrous, was essential in keeping my spirits from sometimes sinking too deep to be reeled back to the surface. Throughout my essays, I mention darkness, blackness, miasma, and, more than once, a dark tunnel. Any caregiver who never finds herself in that dark tunnel knows something I didn't. Laughter brings light into darkness, and I looked for laughter whenever I could find it.

At first I was my only audience to whom I could safely say, "Can you believe this?" After I had gathered a small circle of other caregivers, I'd grab for the phone, bursting to tell someone. Often one of these women would listen, laugh, and then say with painful, rowdy emphasis, "Well, I can top that!" I would listen and laugh in return.

Sometimes I made quick records of conversations with people who undoubtedly meant well. (Actually, I wasn't always so sure about that. I came to adopt a quasi-Freudian attitude toward these supposed well-wishers.) "Today," I once e-mailed Louise, a caregiving friend, "I agreed to meet a former neighbor, newly divorced, for a quick cup of coffee. Bad idea. Dianne talked the whole time about herself and her problems. As we were about to part, she said, 'Oh, and how is James doing? Do you know yet when you'll need to put him in a nursing home?'"

I found in my notes a later and longer anecdote about Dianne, who unknowingly gave me another chance to laugh (outside her hearing). Again to Louise: "On the subject of 'a new life,' which a few people I know have mentioned to me as gloriously awaiting me in the future (as if I would have decades to enjoy it), and I resist spitting in their eyes, I had a hilarious remark aimed at me today. Remember Dianne? Did I tell you she is just about my age, a pretty redhead, very concerned about keeping up her looks? She even had a totally unnecessary face-lift some months ago. Now, in an odd way, she looks rather stretched.

"Anyway, I met her in the grocery store. I know she had a knee replacement a few months ago, so I asked how she was doing. I got a lengthy answer. She asked about me; I said I was more tired than ever. Then I complimented her on looking quite beautiful (which she did, just a little stretched) in an expensive jogging outfit, and she called cheerily to me as I pushed my cart down the aisle, 'Well, Susan, someday *you* will look that way too!'"

I ended such e-mails with one line: "I ask you!"

Sometimes I reacted with both anger and laughter. Writing about those incidents diffused my anger (most of the time) and forced me to salvage a little humor (sometimes). Irony was an essential balm. Just before I took my nine-day break, I spoke with an old friend who lived in a distant suburb. We seldom met. In very different earlier lives, we had known each other well. After this conversation, I understood we no longer did. "I called Josie today," I wrote in my notes. "When I told her I was taking a break next week, her response was, 'Will James be all right?' This reminded me instantly of my mother's asking, so many decades ago, when I was divorced and going out on a rare date, 'What about Jennifer?' My daughter was about three. Of course I had a babysitter. I retorted, 'Oh, I'll just put her in the basement with a bowl of cat food.'

"So I replied to Josie very civilly, all things considered. But I was secretly livid. I told her two of James's children would alternate staying the nights, with Martha handling the days. I wanted to say, 'Of course I don't *know* he'll be all right. I don't know from minute to minute if he'll be all right!'"

(I did not call Josie again for a very long time.)

One of my favorite absurdities involved Martha, our loyal and loving aide. "Martha just knocked on my study door to tell me that when she asked James (very groggy, lying in bed half-awake) how he was feeling, he said, 'I'm feeling sexual.' Martha thought I ought to know. I looked at her blankly. So, she went on, she had plucked a CD called *Saxophone for Lovers* from a pile on the table, and she put that on. She said it calmed him down." Indeed, when I went downstairs, James had gone back to sleep. I have never thought of saxophones the same way since.

I mordantly treasured a birthday card I received as James began his final steep decline. The sender knew very well what was happening, but, upheld by her religious beliefs, she always fervently believed in being positive. Inside was this handwritten message: "Hope your birthday is the beginning of a year where you discover wonderful new directions on your life's path!"

Sometimes the most healing humor was when I could laugh at myself. I immediately think of Rabbit. In "Sleeping with a Wombat," I wrote about my childlike yearning for a large, white plush rabbit I saw in a gift-shop window. One day I bought it. I found it incredibly comforting, something to hold on to at night.

What I found funny is that long after I had written about Rabbit, it turned out not to be a rabbit at all. One of my aides, Trish, once saw me plumping up my stuffed animal and plopping it back onto my pillow. "I love this rabbit," I said somewhat de-fensively. (Women pushing seventy probably aren't supposed to sleep with stuffed animals.) "It's so squeezable." She looked a little more closely.

"But Susan," she said. "That isn't a rabbit. It's a sheep."

"No, no," I replied sternly. "It's a rabbit. I *know* it's a rabbit."

"Sorry about this," she said, starting to smile, "but it's a sheep. See, it doesn't have long ears. The ears are short. Like a sheep. It's round and plump. It has a woolly coat. Like a sheep."

I followed her gaze. Trish was right. Yes, she was definitely right. All these months I had been sleeping not with a rabbit, but a sheep. This was disconcerting. I had nothing against sheep. In fact, during James's and my travels in the U.K., we had spent lots of time around sheep, from hikes through pastures to attendance at sheepdog trials. Sheep were okay—but they weren't lovable. Not like Rabbit.

"Well," I said to Trish, "it is too late for me to change my mind completely about this. I suppose you're right . . ."

"Actually, I am," she said, now smiling quite broadly.

"So," I continued, "I'll just call it Sheepit." From then on, Trish and I occasionally teased each other about my Sheepit. (I secretly continue to call it Rabbit. And I still sleep with Rabbit at night.)

More than four years before James died, when he was still fairly well, I had a revelation that I would need every bit of humor I could find. It was one of many turning points. Unlike my other brief notes, this turned into an undated, longer journal-like entry. I include it here because it conveys something of my typical care-giving day—a mix of love, gratitude, worries, complaints, fatigue, laughter, and, at the very end, a sense of peace. What follows is "His Head Was in the Pansies."

I took James to the dentist for a root canal this morning. He is very good about this, doesn't complain, makes only a small face at the prospect, doesn't fuss and groan as I do. Actually, the morning began with my getting up fairly early, cooking oatmeal and the usual two breakfasts of tea/coffee, juice, two different versions of toast, getting dressed, getting James dressed. Then I had two hurried consultations—one with a plumber about the bathtub drain he was supposed to have fixed yesterday but still leaks—and the other with Blair, painter and Renaissance man, so I could give him a laundry list of painting and repairing tasks he may begin tomorrow.

In the midst of this, Fiona (the housecleaner) arrived to pick up a check for $80—even though she won't come to clean until Thursday—because she wants to go with a girlfriend to Mystic Lake Casino tomorrow. I of course wish she weren't gambling her money away, but I say nothing. She sits down at the table with a glass of lemonade (she has helped herself from the fridge while I was outdoors with Blair) to wait for her bus. These are all too many people for me to cope with. My head hurt when I woke up, and it hurts more now.

Off we go to the endodontist (what IS an endodontist?), arriving promptly at 10:00 a.m. I wait until Dr. Estonia—tall, gangly, and jokey—has come in, looked at the X-rays, and pronounced it okay for me to take a walk while he works on James. Outside it is a totally gorgeous day. I discover behind this block of buildings a winding lake path I had never suspected was here. (What a miracle! I treasure discoveries like these.) Along the path, in the middle of a commercial zone with shops above this sunken level, are purple azaleas in full bloom, crab apples in pink and white glory, carefully chosen trees in different shades of spring green and dark evergreen, nooks with swings for adults, rock gardens, daffodils. I walk for almost forty-five minutes, all around the little hidden lake. I even look assessingly at the large condo developments that edge the lake, those with small (very small) balconies looking out at the water. Maybe someday.

Back in the dental office—I have such a nasty headache today,

*quelled earlier with medication but now starting to reemerge—
I'm told that James has left the chair to go to the toilet. I am a
little concerned about this. I walk out into the hall and circle the
area, since I know where the men's room is. I use the women's
room. Back to the office: I say, "If he doesn't come out in five
minutes, can you send a man in to see if he's okay?" The woman
at the desk says she will. I wait outside in the hall for five minutes. Then I see a young man wheeling a cart of deliveries. I ask
him, and he enters the tiny men's room. "Is James in here?" he
calls. Nope.*

*Now I'm worried. I go back to the office. James has reap-
peared. Everything is fine. I can come back in another fifteen
minutes. (It turns out that when he had to pee, he made this
known—he later described with eloquent gestures how hard this
was with all the apparatus in his mouth—and the doctor had
ushered him into the tiny restroom within the office itself. He
had never been in the hall at all.)*

*So, okay, we get home. I fix James a shake of Häagen-Dazs
chocolate ice cream—he is adamant he doesn't want strawberry,
which I'm pushing because I have some strawberry Ensure to
sneak in—so I find a bottle of chocolate Something Else, an alter-
native Ensure product that tastes like chalk, but the ice cream
will disguise it. He has a glass with a straw: drink, drink it all,
I command. I have a fast turkey wrap I picked up at the pleasant
little café by the lake. Thinking ahead.*

*After lunch I suggest a nap for James. He says he wants to
go outdoors, and no wonder: we've had rain for three days, and
the sun is shining blissfully. So I slap some sunscreen on him,
find his hat, take him out to our tiny backyard patio. Just last
week I bought two oval containers of blooming pansies, bright as
flags, the only flowers that can withstand Minnesota cold/hot/
cold springs. When I look out a few minutes later, he is sitting in
one of our two chairs. The pansies are glinting in the sun. Fine.*

So I call my friend Dolores, and we have a long, companion-

able talk. As I'm talking, I walk to the window. I gasp. James has decided he'd like to lie down. So he has lain flat on the wood planks of the patio and pillowed his head in the middle of one of my containers of pansies. "My God, Dolores!" I say. "I have to hang up. James's head is in the pansies!" I explain; she laughs for a long time and tells me I have to write this down. I say I will. Then I go outside. I am carrying two pillows.

James is asleep. He looks quite touching, lying there in the sun, his head in the flowers. I shake him a little. "James! James! Please, can you move and put your head on these pillows? Your head is in my pansies!" Then we have one of those off-the-wall Parkinson's conversations.

"What are you talking about? My head is NOT in your pansies!"

"Yes, it is! Just sit up, turn around, and look! See where you've smashed the pansies!" Already I'm thinking, why did I start this? Why didn't I say to hell with the pansies?

"No, I don't see it. My head wasn't there."

"Yes, it was. Anyway, just slide a little farther, let me stick these pillows under your head—yes, that's it—and put the hat over your face so you don't get sunburned. Okay? And keep your head out of my pansies!"

A little later he comes back inside. I turn on the latest episode of West Wing, *which he missed last week. It is hard to think of things that will keep him occupied. Right now I need to go downstairs and start dinner. Then I'll set up his iPod to some lovely Robert Shaw Chorale music. This is good.*

Rereading my entries, I saw how much help I had received, sometimes from unlikely people and places. When an overseas friend wrote to ask if I believed in angels (which she did), this is how I answered:

"I have no problem believing in angels, though of course they aren't always there when you wish they were, or maybe they are, and they aren't supposed to intervene or something. Life is a mystery within mysteries, and as long as no one sticks a dogma on top of one of the mysteries, I'm fine with belief. Did I tell you I frequently invoke the images (and angelic presences) of Edgar, James's father (long dead before I knew him, but I feel as if I did, a joyful, generous man with a drinking problem, adored by his son), and my own father Edward, dead at the age of thirty-nine when I was seven? Edgar and Edward, I say, what the hell should I do *now*? Or, Edgar and Edward, how long are you going to let this (whatever it is) go on? Sometimes I get answers, I think, though mainly I just feel comforted by the sense of these two loving male presences.

"On the other hand, it is my handful of women friends (like you) who help me survive."

I needed all the help I could get.

NO SAINTS AROUND HERE

February 19

This morning, tired from a broken night's sleep troubled by bad dreams, I was not in a good mood. So when I had to get up from the breakfast table three times to reheat James's coffee, I soon became snappish. "I wish," I said snidely, in a martyred tone that I learned (alas) from my mother, "you would try to drink your coffee before it gets cold so I wouldn't have to jump up and down like a jack-in-the-box."

James did not respond. He never snaps back. I silently scolded myself as I walked to the microwave. Of course I know he thinks slowly now, he eats slowly, he doesn't remember to drink his coffee. None of this is his fault. He has Parkinson's with dementia. What has happened to me?

I try to forgive myself. I did make my special whole-grain pancakes for him. I pulled over a floor lamp so he could look at the newspaper more clearly. I folded the newspaper to a readable size. I put on his "apron," which is what we call a longish bib, and pushed him carefully into the table. I made sure he had all his pills, water, Kleenex. I'm not an unfeeling spouse. I'm just not a saint.

This morning's irritability was not a rare instance of my failing at sainthood. I sigh a lot. I don't mean inner sighs, but audible, listen-to-me sighs that clearly signal *I am fed up* or *I can't believe this!* or *How can you ask that?*

Maybe James only asked for a glass of water, but I had just opened a letter I wanted to read, right now. Maybe he is taking a short nap, and after doing dishes and emptying garbage, I have just lain down on the other sofa. But no sooner do I put my head on the pillow than James raises his own head. "Is there a basketball game on?" he asks. Never mind that this is Monday afternoon, no playoffs scheduled, maybe a small-town high school team playing somewhere, but certainly not on cable. He doesn't know that.

He is awake, and I have to get up. He needs attention, a move off the sofa, something to do. I heave a THERE-GOES-MY-NAP sigh. Oh, yes, James hears those sighs. Mostly they pass over him, like a short, sharp breeze, and he does not seem to notice. Or he may look up, briefly puzzled, and look at me as if he doesn't understand why I am sighing. And he probably doesn't. But sometimes, when he sees my face, my eyes closing for a second (OH, NO! HOW COULD THIS BE HAPPENING?) and my voice taking on that awful forbearing tone (CAN YOU SEE I'M GRITTING MY TEETH RIGHT NOW?), he'll say, with a brief moment of recognition, "I'm sorry." Then, of course, I feel terrible.

I have a shelfful of books that help me feel guilty. Soon after James was diagnosed, I bought books about Parkinson's. After the first book or two, I didn't find them very useful. I have learned that everyone's Parkinson's is different, something our neurologist confirms. Some sufferers cope with jerky movements, tremors, and freezing episodes when their bodies refuse to move. Others have minor tremors but major mental losses. Some lose their voices; others hallucinate. Some contract the disease fairly young and die quickly, while others last for astonishing decades. Nothing is predictable.

I also began acquiring books about caregiving. One friend, who is interested in the spiritual component of health, brought me several volumes she thought might be useful. They had titles like—not exactly—*The Rewards of Caregiving, A New Commitment, Love All the Way,* and *How Caregiving Made Me a Better Person.*

After dutifully plowing through them, I became more depressed. Many of these writers seemed determined to remind me of my flaws. I frequently failed to concentrate on the beauty of each passing moment. I thought too much about the future. I didn't meditate enough.

I began buying memoirs by caregivers who had taken care of their aging parents, a father with Alzheimer's, a mother with terminal cancer, story after story in which the author learned to combine unselfishness and self-knowledge. Pain and suffering soaked these pages, but peace and enlightenment usually descended in the end. (Of course, in the end, the cared-for person died.)

Finally I found a book that made me feel normal. *The Selfish Pig's Guide to Caring,* by Hugh Marriott, also made me laugh. Marriott is British, and in his country the word "carer" substitutes for "caregiver." Marriott won my heart with his own word coinage. Pondering how to refer to the carer's cared-for-one (and how awkward is that?), he came up with an acronym: the "Person I Give Love and Endless Therapy To" becomes, charmingly, one's "piglet." He does not use "piglet" in a demeaning sense, but with love and humor. My favorite chapter is "Pushing Them Down the Stairs," in which he discusses what to do when a carer, in exhaustion and frustration, has a moment in which he or she wants to do just that.

Marriott reassuringly points out that none of us is a selfish pig. We wouldn't be caregivers if we were. We'd have stashed our loved ones in institutions long ago, called in relatives to take over, maybe changed our names and fled the country. I care for my James not out of duty or obligation but because I cannot yet bear to think of him taken from our home. I'm giving this my best shot. I'm just not a saint.

TOGETHER

February 22

At unexpected times, when I'm doing a task that I may not even find all that onerous, James will say, clearly and with feeling, "You are my hero!" I throw my arms around him. He recently told me, "I can't thank you enough for what you do for me," a whole and coherent sentence. Those words lifted my steps up and down many, many more stairs. Someday he won't be able to say that, and I'll just have to remember when he did.

I don't know how caregivers endure who, before their unrelenting caregiving began, did not have a happy marriage. I met Marcia, now in her late seventies, when she was briefly visiting a friend here. We all had lunch together. Marcia had nursed her husband Tad at home for seventeen years of Parkinson's. Tad had refused—flatly, stubbornly, angrily—to have anyone but Marcia care for him. They had no children. The whole burden fell on Marcia. Marcia's only support was her church, where she had taken her marriage vows, in sickness and in health, with unshakable seriousness.

I could understand all this, but what I couldn't grasp was how she continued to care for Tad after the difficult years of marriage that preceded his illness. I listened to anecdote after anecdote as Marcia told me how Tad had dominated her, his refusal to consider adoption, his unpredictable temper, his dislike of travel, on and on. I found myself asking her what so many well-intentioned friends ask me, "Why didn't you consider a nursing home?"

"Tad wouldn't hear of it," she said simply.

I have been graced. I don't know many people with truly happy marriages. My own first marriage in my twenties failed after a dozen increasingly difficult years. Then I was alone for over a decade, convinced I'd never marry again. Meeting and marrying James in my early forties felt like a miracle. Our twenty-eight years together, even before Parkinson's, weren't always smooth; we had blips and bumps and some bruises as well.

But we took great pleasure in each other's company. We talked together about everything, large and small, and we laughed a lot. In our altered life now, I think I miss most that easygoing, shared laughter. We were both curious by nature. If one of us said, "Maybe we should try that out? Or go here, or there?" the other usually agreed that this was a splendid idea. If one of us suggested, "Why don't we take a chance and turn down that road?" off we went into the unknown.

As an unspoken foundation, we shared fundamental values, planks firmly laid so long ago that we never had to look down to see where they were. (If one of us got off track, the other noticed and called attention.) We had respect for each other's integrity and work. We never lost our physical attraction.

If I have a hard time these days remembering how lucky we really were—and as James dwindles and fades, and I grow more tired and despairing, I do need to remember—I only have to think of the two of us in the front seat of a car. We traveled often. Alone together, as James drove—I had supreme confidence in his driving—I leaned as far over as bucket seats would allow, my head on his shoulder or (if my neck started to hurt) my left hand firmly on his thigh. Of course, occasionally it rained, but in my memory, the sun is bright. I am half-dozing in the warm light flooding through the windshield, my hand feeling James's warmth as well.

"Isn't it time for you to consider a nursing home?" How can I answer? I can't explain all this to anyone, not those twenty-eight years in the detail they deserve, the unwavering support, the wounds given and bound up, the conversation and the laughter. "Wouldn't James, if he could have foreseen what would happen, want you to have a less stressful and exhausting life?" That is an unanswerable question. But it is irrelevant.

RED FLAG IN THE MAILBOX

February 26

Several signs alert me when I'm nearing the edge. Most are predictable—noticing an especially sharp tone when I talk to James, feeling my head throb at the end of the day, wanting so desperately in the morning to stay in bed that I have to invent a heartening reason to get up: "If I push off the covers and set my feet on the floor right now, I could have a quiet half-hour with the newspaper while James is still sleeping."

I can tell I've entered a danger zone when, like today, I open the mailbox and find four small, squished packages among the usual bills, circulars, and appointment reminders.

I know what these packages are. Last week, after I'd tucked James into bed at 7:30 p.m., and I was snugly in my bathrobe, teeth brushed, chores done or postponed, but not quite ready to sleep, I was too tired to read. I usually read under almost any circumstances, at any time, but that night I couldn't bring myself to focus sustained attention on the printed word. I didn't want to watch a DVD or recorded TV program. I couldn't stand to hear any more voices.

Up I went to my computer. Mindlessly, I checked my e-mail. Nothing new. But wait! Right there on my bookmark bar was a magic tab: eBay. I clicked.

I knew I did not need anything. (This is not one of those days when I actually had to find a source for a medical supply or a replacement bedspread or a nonslip rug pad.) My closet is jammed. I live close to several consignment shops so I can scavenge there for anything I want, and until this moment I didn't think I wanted anything.

Now, however, I am seized with a feeling of wanting something. What can I imagine wanting? Maybe I'll just make a few more clicks—like "silk shirt"—and see what's offered. Then I'm plunged into a pictorial feast: red shirts, purple shirts, animal-print shirts, indescribable print shirts.

I don't really plan to buy anything. So I shouldn't be doing this. But I spot a gorgeous blue-and-purple plaid shirt, just perfect over a T-shirt with my jeans. The auction is ending in six hours! No one has bid yet! Of course I'll be in bed when this listing closes, but that doesn't matter. I'm sure I won't win anyway, especially if I put in a low bid—just pennies above the initial price—but what fun if I *did* win! Only eight dollars (and let's not count shipping). I type; I click. I am the high bidder!

And look! Just below that listing is another, and I can so easily see myself in that rosy-pink color, also excellent with jeans. That auction closes minutes after the one I just bid on. Suppose I don't win the first shirt? Should I stake a claim on the second?

Before long I am scrolling, enlarging pictures, mentally trying on shirts and discarding them—or not—and thinking, "What the hell!" as I make another offer, another click.

For half an hour I troll around the site, totally engaged, as if I were so much younger and once again on a shopping spree with a close friend at the after-Christmas sales. We used to "go shopping." I can't believe I ever did that, but I did. We'd set out for the largest local mall, browse in and out of stores, look for bargains, try stuff on, give each other advice. At the end of an afternoon, we'd load up our treasures and congratulate each other on our hunting skills.

I happily shopped with my mother too. She firmly believed that if anything was reduced to 50 percent off, it was our moral duty to buy it. And 70 percent off the retail price? Or even more? Grab it! I still periodically have to purge my closet of dirt cheap items that never even had the utility of a good garden bed of dirt.

I've learned a lot since then. I worry now about money in a way I didn't when I was single and earning a salary, though I always budgeted carefully and never went into debt. I followed *Consumer Reports* faithfully and chose "Best Buys." Now long retired, I am even more careful.

At 9:30 p.m., though, on this particular night, I feel liberated and reckless as I cruise among multicolored silk shirts. I have temporarily blanked out James, in the nearby bedroom, muttering in his half-sleep. I don't remember the tracked-in mud on the hall floor, the bills waiting to be paid, James's bell that will wake me in the middle of the coming night. I need to forget everything for just a little while. More than a glass of wine gives me a headache. I won't be reaching for a bottle. So I click and bid.

That's why, a week later, I know what is in those four packages in the mailbox: a temporary oblivion, a surrender to materialism, a source of yet more guilt. But I do have four lovely shirts costing less than two hours' worth of home help. A good trade? Maybe. Tomorrow, when I need a reason to get out of bed, I'll think of that rosy-pink shirt (practically new, only slightly worn, a very small stain on the cuff).

HIS COLD, MY COLD

March 1

When James began sniffling ten days ago, my heart sank. Yes, I was worried about what a cold might mean for his damaged immune system, but I was also concerned about myself. When my daughter Jenny was a toddler in day care, I dreaded the afternoons when she would run to meet me, and I could see her nose was dripping.

"That's it," I would tell myself morosely.

Two days later, and my own nose would be running like a broken fire hydrant. Sometimes the virus waited three or four days. Sometimes I even became hopeful I'd escape it. But I never did. Jenny got sick, then I got sick, and as a single parent (beginning when she was two), I had no choice but to trudge onward. If anyone dared suggest, "Be sure to drink plenty of liquids, and get lots of rest," I snorted. A snotty, snarky, plugged-up sort of snort.

How did James get his cold? One of my caregivers told me she had warded off a little cold (but she hadn't). Of course, if James and I had remained in isolated hibernation for the entire winter—a thought like jumping hand in hand into a glacial crevasse—I might have murdered him, but he wouldn't have gotten a cold.

The second morning of James's cold I got scared. He awoke

very flushed, more confused than usual, and groggy. I took his temperature: 100°F. Naturally this was Saturday morning, our clinic closed, and our family doctor on a week's vacation. (I remember when Jenny as a child got really sick, she always picked a weekend. The doctor on call, who didn't phone back for hours, usually didn't know who she was.) I dosed James with two extra-strength Tylenol and tried to get him to drink liquids. He hates water. I've never known anyone else who thinks water is yucky, but he does. He'll take a sip grudgingly, but not two sips in a row. He's not fond of fruit juices, tea, or soda, either.

James slept much of the day. I nervously watched him for alarming signs, a higher fever, maybe convulsions, difficulty breathing. I wasn't even quite sure what I should watch for. This was how I'd felt as a single parent, all alone in the middle of the night, watching my child and not knowing what I'd do if she got much worse or what "worse" might be. A caregiver by definition is like a single parent. She's on her own. While I monitor James's cold and downheartedly contemplate my own, undoubtedly lurking in the corner, I think about death. I do this rather often. Parkie—we use that as a shorthand to pretend we're casual about it—is a tricky disease. Parkinson's patients don't usually die directly of Parkinson's. I've read the obituaries: mostly they cite "complications of Parkinson's disease" or state merely that John Smith "had suffered from Parkinson's for twenty years." The words "brave," "courageous," and "struggle" occur, as they do in obituaries mentioning cancer. From my reading and a few queries to doctors, I've learned that James might someday have trouble swallowing and choke to death. (This difficulty in swallowing could explain his aversion to liquids, but he has disliked water for years.)

He might lose his balance, fall, and break a hip. "A bad fall," our Parkinson's specialist has lectured us, "usually means the patient is never the same afterward. We want to avoid falls." Yes, we do, but maybe we can't. James might have a stroke. He might acquire a spreading infection—maybe from a cold, like the one he has now—that could develop into something his immune system could not handle. I won't know until it happens.

James's cold is better now. More than a week later, he is still very tired and easily bewildered. Yesterday, after I'd returned from grocery shopping and a stop at the bank, I found him sitting at the dining table with Martha, our aide. He looked surprised, though very pleased, to see me. When I gave him a quick hug, he said, haltingly, "Oh, so you didn't go to play basketball after all?" I've never played basketball in my life. These moments come and go, but they are apt to appear more often when he is tired or, in this case, recovering from a cold.

Meanwhile my own cold has bloomed. I don't know where I first heard that metaphor, but it is not as peculiar as it first sounds. My cold was not nipped in the bud. Instead it grew within three days into a large, black, monstrous blossom, rather like the titan arum, known as the corpse flower, whose odor is outstandingly repellent to humans because it resembles the stench of rotting flesh. Yes, that's overreaction. After all, with nose spray, I can usually breathe. I apply Mentholatum with a trowel every quarter hour. I take antihistamine. I keep a box of Kleenex in every room. I drink lots and lots of water. I feel miserable, but I know I'm not yet corpse material.

I try to practice positive imagery. I imagine myself tucked up in a large bed, beneath a newly washed, blindingly white, old-fashioned chenille bedspread. A reading light hovers unobtrusively near the bed. On the bedside table is a small, select pile of books, a few novels I've been wanting to read, mostly memoirs, perhaps about becoming a surgeon or trekking in the Arctic or living on a Welsh sheep farm.

Every so often, the landlady knocks gently on the door and brings in a tray with freshly brewed tea, milk, lemon, and honey, as well as a small plate of cinnamon sugar cookies just out of the oven. Later she'll carry up homemade chicken noodle soup, which I have smelled (even with my cold) simmering for hours on the downstairs stove. Apple dumplings for dessert? Or nutmeg-sprinkled custard?

I don't get much further in my fantasy than chicken soup and custard because I have to start thinking about what I'll fix James and myself for supper. No matter how bad my cold, I have to put something tempting on the table at 6:00 p.m. Then I'll get James into his pj's and start his bedtime routine. An hour or so afterward, I'll take another antihistamine, a whiff of nasal spray, something for my headache, and climb into the bed next to his. I hope he doesn't wake too much. I don't have an aide tonight.

Once in bed, I'll turn my noise machine on low and listen to the rhythmic splash of electronic surf. Then I'll pretend I hear a gentle knock on the door, maybe my imaginary landlady bringing me a cup of hot cocoa and ginger biscuits.

LET ME COUNT THE WAYS

March 6

I hate filling pills. Toward the end of every third week—that's how long I can juggle our variously dated prescriptions—I notice that it is time to refill our pillboxes. Time, again.

I used to measure time quite differently. That was before Parkinson's sank its grip so tenaciously into James. How many weeks until a long-anticipated vacation? Days until I concocted a new recipe for a little dinner party? Hours until we could contentedly close the door of our bedroom?

Time has warped now. How can those three weeks have disappeared so quickly? Didn't I do this a few days ago? Or last week? Sometimes I look in the dish cupboard, where I store the piled-up, filled pillboxes, to see if maybe I'm wrong, if maybe another week's worth of pills is sitting there, somewhere I hadn't noticed. Perhaps I put a stack behind the plates? On the bottom shelf by the teabags?

No. I could have sworn we had another week's allotment, but we don't. It is definitely, undeniably, time to fill the pills. In that instant, I become short-tempered. If James interrupts me when I'm counting pills, I will probably answer crossly. Sometimes he says, sweetly and half seriously, ignoring his shaky hands and foggy memory, "Do you want me to do that, Susan?" Ashamed of myself, I roll my eyes and shake my head. If the phone rings or the doorbell buzzes, I swear, quietly but viciously.

I wait for an hour when James is napping, reading, or watching television. I also need to choose an hour when I'm alert—not too late in the day, definitely not after dark. I've been known to forget one or another medication until the boxes have been filled, each little daily tab has been snapped into place, each box covered with a strip of masking tape to prevent accidental spills, each separate stack put away. Then I really swear. James looks alarmed, and I apologize, but I am still filled with inchoate rage as I rip off the tape and prepare to refill.

Filling pills always takes an hour. Sometimes more, never less. An hour. And surely I spend hours every day doing other repetitive tasks, making beds, doing laundry, emptying wastebaskets, carrying out trash, cooking, washing and putting away dishes— whatever. Why should this one task rile me so? It seems so simple, so routine. First I dig out twelve empty pillboxes, each with seven little cavities, from a kitchen cupboard. I line them up on the dining room table. Three are labeled "JAMES MORNING," three "JAMES EVENING," three "SUSAN MORNING," and three "SUSAN EVENING." (I also take several medications and supplements.)

I have labeled each box with the pills that need to go into it, different ones for morning, different ones for night. Several times in the past few years, either rushed or weary beyond carefulness, I have given one or both of us the morning meds at night or the night meds at morning. More than once, I have taken his pills, or he took mine. This is not pleasant. So I try to pay close attention to which pill goes into which box.

Now I retrieve from their shelf all the bottles with nonprescription pills, the vitamins and supplements, the aspirin, the stool softener. I line them up on the table like a battalion of soldiers. These are the less troublesome pills, large and easy to handle. I pour a handful into my palm and count silently—one, two, three, four, five, six, seven—as I pop each pill into its slot.

Sometimes I play a little game with myself, pretending I'll have good luck that day if I've poured out the right number: seven or fourteen or twenty-one.

Even with these pills, though, I can slip and make a mistake. Slippery smooth pills fall through my fingers, dump themselves twice into one slot, or rattle onto the table. I've learned to keep a table knife next to the boxes so I can use it to pry out pills that land in the wrong slot.

When I have finished with the nonprescription pills, I stand up and stretch. Almost halfway through. Now comes the harder part: the prescription pills. If I miss a calcium tablet, no big deal. But if I skip James's antacid or antidepressant, his life might hit a minor bump that day. And if I forgot a week's supply of any of our prescriptions, the bump might turn into a pothole.

I separate the pill bottles, his and mine, on two sides of the table. I have to make sure that his twice-a-day ones go into both "Morning" and "Evening." As I fill the boxes, sometimes I see that I'm running out of pills. Efficient as I am, with a computer program to remind me of refills, occasionally a prescription refill date eludes me. So I'll fill the rest of his pills and put a Post-it note on each box: MISSING ACIPHEX. I place the empty bottle on the kitchen counter; I'll call the drugstore as soon as I'm done. I'll also stick a Post-it on my kitchen window, which serves as another desktop: WALGREEN'S.

By the time I am ready for my own pillboxes, I can feel accumulated stress in my neck and shoulders. I stand, wiggle, and shake. Since I'm up, I'll tackle the potassium, a giant horse pill impossible to swallow comfortably. I have to split it in two. But even the biggest pill splitter I've found can't quite handle it. The pill crumbles into two uneven, powdery, grainy halves. I operate with a sharp knife on a wooden cutting board (thinking, peripherally, about the bacteria undoubtedly hovering there), so I can sweep all the potassium residue away with my dishrag.

The last part of pill filling goes quickly. I drop all the split pills into their slots with a sense of satisfaction. Plop, plop, plop. Then I snap the daily lids shut, very, very carefully. Once, not long ago, I was so exhilarated to be done that I snapped those lids with too much exuberance. That weekly pillbox jumped, as if startled, and emptied itself onto the table, and as it jumped, it knocked against a second pillbox, which also spilled an undifferentiated heap on the table. I think I screamed, which really alarmed James.

On another pill-filling day, I had all twelve boxes complete but still open when one of our three cats suddenly leaped onto the table. She swiftly swooshed all twelve pillboxes off the table, scattering pills onto the dark complicated patterns of our Oriental rug, where, on my hands and knees, I had to squint to see them. This time I know I screamed. I may have grabbed for the cat. She wisely ran upstairs.

Now I am very, very careful. After closing all the lids, I affix a strip of masking tape to each box with a firm but cautious touch. The stash for this week goes onto the kitchen counter, and I slide the rest into the dish cupboard. Before I put them away, however, I stand up and admire them, those neat stacks of pillboxes, medicines counted and apportioned, three weeks of safeguards for the twenty-one days ahead.

I briefly feel a wave of relief, the gentle relaxing of tense muscles that happens when James has fallen into a steady sleep on the sofa, or when the door has closed behind him as one of his children has taken him to an afternoon movie, or when I pour myself a second cup of tea at breakfast and, checking my video monitor, see that James shows no signs of waking up yet. Three weeks of pills filled: a task done. Almost three weeks until the next time.

Then another, less welcome wave laps darkly at my relief. Is this how the rest of my life will be, as I too grow into old age and decrepitude? I love this man profoundly, but still, I wonder. Will I be measuring the coming years like this, filling pills, until someday, when I myself am helpless, someone else has to fill them for me?

Sometimes as I put away all the pill bottles and the filled boxes, I think of a line from "The Love Song of J. Alfred Prufrock": "I have measured out my life in coffee spoons." I first read Eliot's poem at seventeen. "Prufrock" was such a cautionary tale. At seventeen, I wanted to measure life in gulps, in swaths, in romances, in unreeling adventures. I remind myself that over the years, I have indeed measured it in many of those ways. Now I measure it in pills. I am trying to think of Eliot's verse as part of a continuing love song.

FAILING BATTERY

March 10

A caregiver needs to make plans, but she should always make them in disappearing ink.

Yesterday morning, remembering that my aide Martha would soon come for several hours, I thought, "Hey! After I've driven to the grocery store, the bank, and the mall to order new bifocals, I might still have time for a quick walk." In deciding how I could apportion my time, I had, as usual, in George W. Bush's famous coinage, "misunderestimated."

Off I hustled. But when I opened the garage and turned the key in my ignition, I noticed that my dashboard clock had mysteriously reset to 1:00 a.m. The time, according to my watch, which I constantly consult like a nervous twitch in my wrist, was 11:00 a.m. Nor was this the first time the clock had startled me. The day before, and the day before that, I also had turned the key and discovered the time was 1:00 a.m. As I punched buttons to restore the correct hour yet again, I wondered if the clock knew something I didn't. Was I always living in the sleepy murkiness of 1:00 a.m.?

Still, I knew it would be best to consult Tony, my terrific mechanic, whose garage is not far away. Tony, however, was out to lunch, and his assistant told me I should return in an hour. Now

I was half an hour off schedule. The grocery store had long lines. I had a list, but I'd left it in the car. I rolled my cart so fast up and down the aisles that I bumped a few cans of tuna fish off the end-cap display. (That was okay; I decided we needed some tuna fish.) I took too long to choose the right frames for my glasses, because caregiver or not, I still have regrettable vanity. The bank teller, now practically an old friend, and I got into a discussion about why the U.S. Mint no longer prints denominations higher than a hundred-dollar bill. (I wasn't asking for a thousand-dollar bill, but I was longing for a little adult conversation.)

When I finally turned into Tony's lot, I was convinced I'd never get home at the time I'd promised Martha. Tony propped up the hood, and two other mechanics joined him in diagnosing the problem. Soon Tony beckoned me. He pointed to a large device he'd attached to my battery, with numbers he then calculated and reentered. "Your battery is marginal," he said cheerily. No problem. He could fix this, he added, by fiddling with the connections. Just another fifteen minutes.

My battery is marginal. I thought about that. I thought about it all the way home. I was quite tired now. I wouldn't have time to walk. I wished I could take a nap. Yes, like the clock turning over relentlessly to 1:00 a.m., my own battery is definitely marginal.

SLEEPING WITH A WOMBAT

March 16

W hen I flop into my downstairs bed at night, I curl up next to my wombat.

He is much smaller than an ordinary wombat—if wombats, those secretive, nocturnal Australian creatures, can ever be considered ordinary. There is much to be said for sleeping with this wombat. He is utterly tranquil. He doesn't wake or turn uneasily when I get up at night. Although not seductively silky like a cat, his stiff, fuzzy fur is strokable. But sometimes, as I put my arms around him, I'm not always sure which end is which. His rotund pigginess makes it hard to find his tiny ears and small snout. If I'm drifting off to sleep, I can become disconcerted if I find I'm hugging his rear end. I have to turn him around before I can truly fall asleep.

When I don't have a night aide and I sleep upstairs in a bed next to James, I grab the giant-size white rabbit who perches unobtrusively on a nearby chair. I first saw Rabbit several years ago in a gift-shop window, when I was hurrying to my therapist's office. I didn't consult her very often then; James's Parkinson's was still fairly mild. I paused briefly to look at this rabbit, its floppy ears, pink nose, thick white fur, and a sweet expression, almost a half-smile, on its rabbity face. Then I caught myself: "Good grief. This is a *stuffed animal*. Come on. You are *grown up*! You don't have any grandchildren. You don't even *know* a child who would want this rabbit. You have no excuse for buying it. Move along!"

The fluffy white rabbit didn't sell. The next month, I walked tentatively into the gift shop and asked the clerk to take Rabbit out of the window. He curled up in my arms, very soft, very huggable. I didn't want to put him down. On an impulse, I whipped out my credit card. I didn't even try to justify the purchase to myself. When I walked into my therapist's office, carrying a large stuffed animal, I said, a little embarrassed, "I just had to have this." She looked at Rabbit and nodded. "I can see why," she said.

Rabbit is the perfect size for someone who sleeps on her side and wants to wrap her arm around something comforting. He is even more squeezable than Wombat, but if I'm tossing, sleepless, during the night, Wombat reminds me of a relaxed afternoon strolling through the Queen Victoria market in Melbourne, Australia. A few days before I bought Wombat, James had patiently tapped his cane through Melbourne's sprawling, landscaped zoo so I could finally see a real wombat. I had just read a classic naturalist's memoir, *The Secret Life of Wombats,* and I was entranced. Unlike holding Rabbit, when holding my wombat, I am clinging to a lost part of my life.

I did not always yearn for a stuffed animal. I had James.

When we married, we added two large bedrooms onto his bachelor house, one for my teenage daughter Jenny and one for us. James planned ours carefully. We were both restless sleepers, even then, and James was a sleeper with a symphony of noises— snores, snorts, coughs, thunderous farts. Once, when we tried sleeping in the same bed, I woke up terrified in the middle of the night. "James, James!" I whispered urgently, poking him awake. "Someone is in the house! I just heard a gunshot!" James turned over and looked at me sleepily. "No," he said calmly. "That was just me. Go back to sleep."

Our new bedroom didn't have space for two large beds, and James didn't mind sleeping in a twin. So I got a spacious queen next to his smaller one: "Two beds for sleeping, one for sex," he liked to explain slyly to visitors. Most of our house has small rooms, but this one is spacious and lofty, with a high-pitched sky-blue ceiling, a square window cut into it so we can see the sky. From our beds, we look out into treetops, as if we were living in the woods, not in the heart of a city. Light streams in from windows on three sides, bouncing off three crossbeams painted pink, yellow, and blue. It is a joyous room.

We were very happy together in that bedroom. Early in the morning, if I woke first, I would call across to the other bed. James, still mostly asleep, would stumble across the small gap and climb in beside me. Or sometimes I'd wake to find his warm body curled next to mine already.

Now, dispossessed by Parkinson's, whose hallucinatory nightmares have exacerbated James's nighttime awakenings and murmurings into such noisy interruptions that I have had to move downstairs, I still try to spend several nights a week in our bedroom. But Parkinson's has also stiffened James's muscles so that he cannot turn over in bed. He has to sleep all night on his back, sprawled almost crosswise on his twin bed, because once he's prone, I can't center him properly. This in turn means I have no room to slip into his bed. It is a terrible loss.

Even those who know little about art history often are familiar with one famous image from Michelangelo's fresco on the ceiling of the Sistine Chapel. God is reaching out to Adam, who in turn stretches yearningly toward him. Michelangelo has captured the electrifying moment when their fingers almost touch. Humans are created by touch.

I can still touch James, and I do, in as many ways as possible. I can hug him, and, straining, he can awkwardly hug me back. When we sit on the sofa together, watching a DVD, I make sure I have an arm around him. I apply body lotion, and I pat his cheek as I shave him. I get him out of bed, and I tuck him in. He is never far from my hands.

That sense of nearness is what my two friends whose husbands died this year tell me they miss so acutely. "At least he's there," one said recently, after hearing my litany of complaints. "Physically *there*. You have not lost that." The other friend says often, "Treasure this time. Treasure it." Oh, right, I sometimes think sardonically to myself on the hardest days. But I know what she means.

Still, I sleep alone at night. So downstairs I have Wombat, and upstairs I have Rabbit.

Not long ago, walking down an aisle in our very crowded, disorganized mishmash of a drugstore, I spied a huge stuffed polar bear looming over a high shelf of toppling children's games. I have always thought of polar bears with awe, almost as totems, emblems of the fierce mysteriousness of life and death. I wanted that bear.

I asked a passing clerk, who was just tall enough, to lift it down. If it could stand, it would be almost my height. Being soft and plush, it sits and flops, this way and that way, while staring bearishly out at an unknowable landscape. I could not sleep with this bear. It was too big. But I wanted it anyway. It was twenty dollars. I did not hesitate.

The polar bear could not fit in any bag. As I checked out, the cashier smiled when I tucked it under one arm. Its large white head jutted far forward, its ample rear nudged the woman behind me. "So is this bear for a grandchild?" the cashier asked with a smile. "No," I said firmly. "It's for me." People I passed on the sidewalk turned for a moment to watch me carry Polar Bear to my car.

Now Polar Bear has taken over—indeed, almost obliterated—a small table in my downstairs bedroom. Silent but alert, Polar Bear steadily looks toward my door, on guard. When I get up at night to go to the bathroom, I like to see it there, a whiteness faintly shining in the dark.

STUFF, STUFF, STUFF

March 19

Crammed onto our bedroom shelf is a carton of the wrong kind of incontinence products. I keep it because I think someday it might be the right kind. The bulky carton is wedged between an unread biography of Winston Churchill and a P. D. James murder mystery. I didn't know where else to put it.

Caregiving has blown through our house like a small tornado, scattering stuff everywhere. So many boxes of Kleenex litter the rooms—on the coffee table, dining table, sofa, end table—that it seems someone needs to have a tissue constantly within arm's reach. (He does.) A large plaid bib hangs over James's dining room chair. A small wastebasket stands next to the chair.

I can barely find space to lay out two dinner plates on our kitchen counter because I have to make room among weekly pillboxes, daily pill bottles, a calendar for charting doses, a bag of the only crackers that James likes well enough to nibble when he is feeling queasy, and pens and Post-its so I can remember to note recycling day, important phone calls to return, and innumerable to-dos that I scribble in my own code ("Books on stairs," "Sarah," "Bank 20s") and slap on the window over the sink. I am at the sink so often that I use the window as my urgent bulletin board.

I haven't yet mentioned the kitchen countertop box of

Kleenex (of course), a pile of small cans of cat food, a spray bottle to shoo cats, a telephone, and a bottle of baby oil with an eyedropper, which I am supposed to use frequently to soften my earwax, but which I seldom remember to do, so I'm hoping that looking frequently at the bottle will remind me.

I have never been a punctilious, spotless housekeeper. I've known homes—mostly photographs in magazines—that never seem to accumulate magazines, unread copies of the Sunday newspapers, a sweater tossed over the sofa, or a purse flung onto the stairs. They don't display family pictures, colorful or whimsical oddments, or boot trays or mail baskets or rows of DVDs. Even before James's Parkinson's, our house wasn't one of them.

But despite my lack of minimalism, I do like a sense of order. I do not feel easy in a house that isn't basically tidy. If I have books in a pile, it is a neat pile, out of the way of a careless foot. I can't ever leave pots and pans in the sink and plan to wash them in the morning. As I used to explain patiently to James, who wanted me to come to bed when a dinner party was over, "I won't be able to sleep until I get all this cleaned up." I'm an organizer, a woman whose first piece of furniture for her study was a four-drawer filing cabinet.

So adjusting to all the stuff that Parkinson's has brought into our life has not been easy. I can't wish this stuff away, and I can't usually put it away, either. Next to his bed, James needs a clock with oversized numbers, an intercom, a large brass bell, and a glass of water with lid and straw—and (of course) a box of Kleenex. Without moving more than a step, I have to be able in the night to lay my hands quickly on pills, Chapstick, dry-mouth spray, and dry-skin lotion.

Two open canvas boxes take up most of the closest bookshelf. Martha, our aide, needs instant access to cotton balls, assorted creams and gels, razor, antiseptics, thermometer, blood pressure monitor, acetaminophen, and more. When she starts to work on James, gently and tenderly, she likes her tools handy.

The rest of our bedroom is crowded too. Entering the room, no one can miss the commode, a bright blue pseudochair anchored askew to the wood floor (but at the right angle for James, swinging out of bed). To raise the head of his bed, since Parkinson's causes acid reflux, I've installed a large inflatable wedge under James's mattress, which in turn requires an on-floor pump plugged into an extension strip of electric outlets. Under one window is an open canvas basket filled with "gentlemen's pads" and another with extra mattress cover, sheets, and leakproof bedpads. I keep a spare clean set of pajamas on the window seat. In case of need, I too want supplies ready to grab.

Our house is strewn with evidence of what is happening here. Seated in his enveloping, cushioned chair and warned not to try to rise without help, James naturally expects to have several boxes of old pictures, design projects, and mementos of his professional life close enough so he can reach them. He likes a box or two in the living room, too, which I daily put away under the piano. I find loose snapshots here and there on the floor. I pick them up.

Martha plays CDs for James on a clunky, glaringly red portable player (right price, right size) I recently bought for him. In earlier days, James would have insisted I take it right back to the store and find one less resoundingly ugly. But he doesn't seem to notice now, and besides, I have no time to search around for one more aesthetically pleasing. So the CD player hovers in our bedroom, blinking its red light, like a miniature, patched-together spaceship, all bumps, buttons, and awkward curves.

Martha has decided to keep stacks of different music next to the Alien Player so James can decide whether he wants, say, Tommy Dorsey, Mozart, country hits, Hawaiian songs, or the Robert Shaw Chorale. Some days he likes to have a massage while listening to Renée Fleming. Other days it is Willie Nelson. The CDs spill over into a heap.

Everything in the house seems to spill over into heaps. Bed pillows at the end of the sofa so James can nap propped up; a small pile of paper towel segments near his plate, because he prefers those to napkins; mail on the stairs so I can take it up to my desk on my next trip. Sometimes I walk determinedly through our rooms with mental blinders.

A caregiver has almost no time to sort through drawers, cupboards, or shelves. Several weeks ago, fed up with feeling helpless amid so much mess, I emptied our all-purpose kitchen drawer onto our main counter. An assortment of screwdrivers, rubber bands, scissors, keys, paper clips, pliers, tape measures, labels, and more lay on the counter for almost two days. I simply did not have an hour to deal with it all.

Once the drawer was reorganized, however, I was inordinately pleased. I sometimes open and close it now even when I don't need anything from it, just so I can see how neat and ordered it looks. I have one very clean kitchen drawer. Just one.

"Don't sweat the small stuff," James used to tell his children when they were growing up. They fondly mention this. It was excellent advice. Why, then, don't I follow it? Why do I fret about this mess that is an inescapable part of a caregiver's life? Why can't I just let it go?

I think I am actually fretting about loss of control. James and I used to shape our life together, making conscious decisions and compromises. Now Parkinson's has taken our life and violently shaken it, whirling it around with centrifugal fury, forcing bits and pieces to fly off into space. Our core is still there. But we are losing more all the time.

OVERLOADED

March 23

When someone asks me, "How are you doing, Susan?" I often reply, "Overloaded." My questioner nods understandingly, but I'm not sure he or she knows exactly what I mean. This is what I mean:

On my kitchen counter, I keep a tiny vial of Wite-Out, useful for erasing canceled plans and appointments from my wall calendar. Caregivers frequently cancel. I also keep a tiny vial of liquid bandage, since, as I'm scurrying around my kitchen, I frequently nick my finger instead of slicing a carrot. I try to slow down. I try to be careful. But things happen.

This morning, having hurried to get James's breakfast almost ready (he was still asleep), I remembered that I hadn't taken out last night's laundry from the dryer. I was also out of dish detergent. So I scooted down to the basement and piled the heap of dry laundry into a basket. While I was downstairs, I also smelled the fact that the cats' boxes needed emptying. I scooped their leavings into a paper bag and put that on top of the laundry basket. I grabbed a sixteen-ounce bottle of dish detergent and stuck that in the basket too.

But as I hoisted the overflowing basket, the bottle fell out and struck me hard on my anklebone. Really hard. I yelped. Who would have thought an ankle could hurt so much from such a minor jolt? Up in the kitchen again, I looked at my ankle. I saw a very small cut from the flying bottle. How could a plastic container cut through skin? But it did.

Without thinking, I grabbed a small vial and dabbed Wite-Out on the cut. That was when I grasped that not only my basket was overloaded.

THE NURSING HOME
ON THE HILL

March 26

M any of our friends believe I should be heading there today, driving James and his belongings to a nursing home. They seem to picture it as a pleasant, well-lit, homelike place on a hill, surrounded by landscaped grounds and tended by dedicated, sunny nurses, where James will be, eventually, fine. Just fine. Well looked after.

"The adjustment might be difficult," some will admit, "but he would get used to it. It might take some time. And of course you could visit all you want. You wouldn't be deserting him. But you would be free at last. You deserve a life." They pronounce that last sentence almost like a threat.

One advocate encouragingly told me about a friend of hers who'd had a complicated operation and had to recuperate in a nursing home for several weeks. "Gerry actually enjoyed it," my friend said. "She got great care, and she spent the time reading, watching movies, and just resting. I visited her once, and I was really impressed with the level of attention she got."

They don't know. First, I'm not sure they know what the dementia section of a nursing home is really like. A year ago, watching James's cognitive abilities noticeably decline again—they seem to fall sharply, level off, then fall once more—I decided I had better investigate the future possibility of a nursing home. I know that I cannot care for James at home under all circumstances. At some point I may need to concede. I had better be prepared.

I chose two for visits. (I was so disheartened afterward that I decided to postpone my field studies a while longer.) The first was a very large, well-endowed, highly touted complex that offered assisted-living apartments as well as nursing care. Lakeview Manor (which had, as promised, partial views of a small lake) was known as the top choice in our city. Before my guide came to get me, I wandered around a little. The Manor did indeed have a very large open public space, though furnished with the overupholstered, tartan-plaid furniture and Early American coffee tables James loathed. Nobody was sitting in the chairs or on the sofas.

I also couldn't see anyone on the enclosed glass porch overlooking the lake. Perhaps on this winter day the room was too cold. I wondered if James would sit there in the summer. Summer in this part of the world isn't very long.

The whole place was eerily quiet. I poked my head in here and there. No one in the tiny library, either. I checked out the "family dining room," where, my brochure said, its residents—I tried not to think of the word "inmates"—could entertain at private parties. The room was rather claustrophobic and quite dark because it had no windows. Maybe it would look more welcoming with its fluorescent light turned on. Maybe not.

My guide, Alice, perky and informative, showed me through the whole complex. The one vacant assisted-living apartment I saw, though small, looked nice enough, especially if one had few possessions. But when I mentioned that James's Parkinson's had induced a certain amount of dementia, Alice said regretfully, "Then, of course, he couldn't be in this section. You have to be mostly independent to live here. I'll take you up to the Memory Floor."

The Memory Floor was supposed to evoke Parisian street life. Its halls had gay painted murals featuring sidewalk cafés, men in berets on bicycles, and rather demure cancan dancers. Public rooms carried names like "Montmartre" and "Bois de Bologne." Nothing reminded me in the least of Paris.

I saw one nearly empty room. "This resident is moving out today," Alice said. I asked her where this patient was going, and Alice said apologetically she was not legally able to tell me. A locked ward? A funeral home? The room had one high window that included sky and trees, though not easily visible from the bed, and just enough space for a bed, chest of drawers, and an easy chair. Most furniture had been removed, but I am sure the room could also have held a television set and perhaps a bookcase. I thought of our wide, sunny windows at home and rooms where James still enjoyed walking from one to another.

Then Alice took me into the Memory Floor dining area, a bright room with a long table and several chairs. Three old women sat there, one still at the table with a disheveled breakfast tray in front of her. She was looking at her lap. She glanced up when we came in and then looked away, expressionless. "We feed our residents on this floor whenever they wake up and want breakfast," said Alice. It was now noon. The two other women sat in wheelchairs, staring blankly in front of them. They too were expressionless. One of them was drooling a little.

Alice wanted to show me the basement-level exercise room and swimming pool. James wouldn't be lifting any dumbbells or sitting at any machines, and he hated pools. I was longing to flee.

I dutifully sat down with Alice in her office, however, and went through the briefing documents. I checked the basics: initial costs, later costs, additional costs. This would be extra, that would be extra. I was reeling. A few years of this, and we'd be in Medicaid country.

It took several weeks for me to recover from the baleful cloud the Memory Floor had draped over my idea of a nursing home.

Then I steeled myself and arranged another visit, this one to a very small institution, actually a large converted house. Summerfield House catered to only twelve residents. It was an easy fifteen-minute drive from our house, in a moderately upscale residential area just off a freeway. I thought it sounded promising.

If money were not an issue, Summerfield might have been a possibility. The staffing ratio was about one to three residents, the food was often cooked at home by one of the staff, and the house had an outdoor deck overlooking a backyard with lawn and trees. For such intimacy and personal attention, the fees were about what Lakeview Manor cost. Good care is expensive.

But as soon as I entered, I stifled a sigh. Darkness again: renovation, cutting larger spaces into individual rooms, had forced the elimination of many windows. The decorator—"She does all our houses," my Summerfield guide said with an apologetic shrug—had summoned dreary kitsch like a bad fairy. Dusty artificial flowers in vases, banal prints on the walls, brown-and-green color schemes, drab floral cushions. If he left his room, James would have to sit on a plastic-covered sofa and stare at all this.

I saw one large room where I could just, almost, imagine James. It had good light, though because it was below grade level, its band of high windows offered no view. I could move a few pieces of contemporary furniture into this space; here he could breathe. To eat his meals, he would move into a small common space shared with the adjoining room—where, I saw, a huge TV was blaring, although no one was watching it.

Someday environment may not matter to him. That will certainly be one of my signals to consider a move. But environment will still matter to me. "Of course you could visit James every day," my friends assure me. Yes, I could. But when I visited, what would I do? Would I take James upstairs and seat us among the dusty dried flowers, making what conversation we could with the other residents? Would I stay in his room, fasten my iPod headphones onto James's ears and sit, reading, in that confined space? Would we move into the TV room and watch whatever channel someone else had already selected? An old Western? Soap operas? Endless CNN?

At home, at this moment, while he is still relatively mobile and able to communicate, though with difficulty, James doesn't have a staffing ratio of one-to-three. He has one-to-one. Carefully selected helpers (including, at the center, a wife who loves him) give him dedicated attention. If he is bored with music, I can arrange an audiobook. If a DVD disturbs him, he rings a bell, and I can turn it off. When he feels restless, either I or one of my aides can take him for a walk around the house or, in good weather, outdoors.

"You deserve a life." What do my well-meaning advisers think my life would be like if I moved James into a nursing home? I know I would want to visit every day at least as long as he knew who I was. Love, years of incalculable attachment, undoubted guilt: how could I walk away? I have a friend whose husband, with severe Alzheimer's, cannot speak or recognize her, but she drives many miles most days of the week to give him company, feed him, and make sure he is being cared for properly.

How would I feel when I saw James strapped into a wheelchair, perhaps sedated, because no one could be with him every minute to make sure he didn't try to stand up and then fall down? Who would take the time to wash his scalp carefully, gently, every day with a medicated shampoo to alleviate an itchy flakiness that Parkinson's has added to his symptoms? How quickly would he lose more weight when he no longer could be so irritatingly choosy about exactly what he would or would not eat? Who would give him hugs, stroke his face, try to make him smile?

Not long after my visits to Lakeview Manor and Summerfield House, I took James for one of his quarterly visits to our Parkinson's specialist. After his usual checkup, I asked to speak to Dr. Sutton alone. James didn't remark on this. I am sometimes glad there is much he doesn't notice anymore. Quickly, in her private office, I told her that I was still hoping to care for James at home until the end. ("His or yours?" one friend once asked me sardonically.) But, I continued, knowing that the time might come when I could not continue, I had now investigated two nursing homes. I described them both; she knew them well.

Dr. Sutton did not ask whether I had visited any others. Nor did she point out the undeniable fact that many caregivers have to settle, often desperately and agonizingly, for a nursing home with far less agreeable comfort and amenities.

After I had given her my disheartening picture of the blank-faced women on the Memory Floor, the messy breakfast tray, the silence, she nodded in recognition. "Well," she said, pushing her chair back so we could return to James, "then you realize how far James has yet to go."

I hope the Nursing Home on the Hill will remain a distant vision. But I cannot avoid noticing what is happening. Many days it looks as if it has moved closer.

TEETH TORTURE TIME

March 29

When I woke up on Friday, I felt unexpectedly energetic. Then at breakfast James said, haltingly, between slow spoonfuls of Corn Flakes, "I think I have a loose tooth." I was bustling in the kitchen, cleaning up, feeding cats, and looking forward to aide Martha's arrival. But a loose tooth was serious. My promising morning had just developed a nasty blip.

For several years James has suffered from dry mouth. Parkinson's and its medications can do that. Nothing we've tried seems to help. Dry mouth is not only uncomfortable, it is also an open invitation to bacteria and tooth decay. Anyone with dry mouth needs to see his dentist often. Just two weeks ago, James had a checkup (five small new cavities await filling).

After breakfast, while brushing and flossing his teeth, I tried to get James to point to the loose tooth. First he tapped a lower tooth on one side, then, after some hesitation, changed his mind and tapped one on the other side. He wasn't sure. I gently tried to wiggle both possible loose teeth, and I thought maybe, just maybe, I detected a little movement. I sighed to myself. What to do? Another trip to the dentist? So soon? James did feel something was wrong. I should trust that. So I went to the phone and wrangled an emergency appointment. When Martha arrived, I asked her to drive James to our dentist's office. When they returned, Martha was carrying a paper sack, which meant, ominously, Dr. Alder had sent home supplies.

I should explain about my relationship to James's teeth. I didn't used to have one. He went into our bathroom at night and presumably brushed and flossed. I never observed this. Thankfully, we did not have that kind of togetherness. He also went for cleanings that I scheduled twice a year. I planned my own appointments so they coincided with his, so I only had to drive to the dental office once. He had his dental hygienist; I had mine.

But a few years ago, as I was pinned into a dental chair, waiting for our dentist to inspect my newly shining mouth, James's hygienist entered the cubicle. She was carrying a piece of floss and looking at it with palpable distaste.

"James is not flossing at all well," she said accusingly. Dr. Alder and I stared at the floss. We could both see largish bits of dangling food. It was not an attractive sight. "His gums are in terrible shape," she went on. "If he isn't able to take care of his teeth, you will have to start doing it." Then she turned and went back to my errant husband. Dr. Alder looked at me. "Well, Susan, she's right," he said. "From now on, you'd better take charge of that." He peered into my mouth, tested his instruments here and there, and left the room.

Dot, my hygienist, eyed me sympathetically. "Oooh, ish," she said, making a face. "I don't think I could ever floss my husband's teeth." She had echoed my own feelings completely. I eyed her back. I was thinking *oooh, ish* a lot more strongly than she was.

"Tell me something, Dot," I replied. "Do you think Dr. Alder would ever floss *his* wife's teeth?" She didn't hesitate. "Not in a million years," she said decisively.

That wasn't much comfort. I knew all too well that decaying teeth and rotten gums lead to an unpleasant outcome. I did not want James toothless.

James didn't like Dr. Alder's idea either. That night James argued that he was quite capable of brushing his own teeth. I asked him to demonstrate. As I watched, he swished his toothbrush back and forth across his teeth a few times. Five seconds, maybe ten. I noticed how his hand trembled slightly with Parkinson's. I didn't bother to observe his flossing technique. "Okay," I said. "Here's the point." I sucked in my lips with exaggeration as if I were toothless and lisped, "Do you really want to end up looking like this?" He considered. He got the point.

Brushing James's teeth is not easy. He loathes the vibration of his electric brush, mandated by Dr. Alder. As I try to manipulate it up and down, back and forth, front and back, James bobs and weaves, as though he were dodging a swarm of bees. "Stand still!" I snap, as I accidentally jab him in the side of his mouth. He winces. He usually has troublesome dry mouth, but at this moment he is dripping saliva. He rolls his eyes in protest. Then I poke around with a specially ordered set of small flossy picks, all in different sizes to fit into different crevices. He stands fairly still for this, but I have to dodge the flying specks. I'm not always fast enough.

I call this twice-daily process, quite accurately, Teeth Torture Time. Sometimes, to boost my spirits, and maybe James's, I sing defiantly as I brush. I use a tune I remember from long ago on *Howdy Doody*. Someone always introduced this children's show with a cheery musical refrain: "It's Howdy Doody Time!" I carol instead: "It's Teeth Torture Time, oh it's Teeth Torture Time. We're trying to save the teeth, we're trying to save the teeth. We really *hate* all this, we really *hate* all this, but it's Teeth Torture Time." Occasionally this helps.

Many of my duties as caregiver that would sound quite unbearable to someone who hadn't done them are, in fact, no big deal. But I still hate brushing and flossing James's teeth.

So when Martha laid out the contents of the dental sack on our dining-room table, I knew Teeth Torture Time was about to get more complicated. James, it turns out, had not a loose tooth but an abscess. It had developed in his gum almost overnight. Now he would need oral antibiotics three times a day for a week (probably including the middle of the night), and I would have to use a tiny tool, like a miniature mop, to gently dab a prescription mouthwash all around the lanced abscess. Twice a day for three days. Then, with a new and extraordinarily soft toothbrush, I should strive to keep the area spotlessly clean, using the same mouthwash, for two weeks until his next appointment.

James was looking out the window, disinterested. Martha was explaining again what had to be done. I was thinking gloomily that in just a few hours, I would need to brush James's teeth.

TIME ON THE TUNDRA

April 7

I am trudging across an endless, frozen tundra. Everything is blurred into the same numbing color—ice, snow, sky. Pushing a heavy sled ahead of me, its strapped bundles teetering, I cannot see a horizon. I have no idea where I'm going. Time has vanished. I just keep moving.

That was exactly how I felt two days ago, when a brief snowstorm pushed an unbearably long winter even further into April. I did not see myself as an explorer, however, headed toward a new discovery. I was not brave, not adventurous, just stupefied. I was trapped on a journey without map or compass.

A caregiver's routine can sometimes bring on a mental snowstorm. That morning I heard myself give James exactly the same instructions as every other morning. "Okay, grab the white bar, grab the other bar, sit down." At the dining table: "Straight ahead, to the chair, that's right, uncross your legs, pull into the table." I have many such formulaic phrases. "No, not that way, up the stairs. Up the *stairs*. To your closet. Your *closet*." I live in an echo chamber.

I do exactly the same things every morning. Get up promptly at seven—my night aide's duty ends at seven, and I need to give James his pill—and start moving fast. Out of my bed to check on

James. Move him from his bed to commode, back to bed. Dress myself quickly. Downstairs, open front door, take in newspaper. Fix myself a speedy breakfast, all the while watching my video monitor to make sure James has gone back to sleep.

Let the cats out of their room—impossible to permit their jumping up and down on our beds during the night—and feed them. Grab the fat cat, and set her down in a small bathroom so she can't eat the other cats' food. These are not the most wonderful cats I have ever owned, but no one else would want them. So they remain.

Now it is time to set out the morning pills, his and mine. Cut his big ones in half. Place the Kleenex, sheets of paper towel, and wastebasket by his chair. Pour juice and water. Start his coffee. Put away last night's dishes if I had been too tired to do that. Oops, fresh water for the cats. We're almost out of orange juice. Make a note. Oops again, I need to move James's bottle of laxative where I'll see it, or I might forget the morning dose. Uh oh, James is now moving again, antsy, wanting to start his day. Upstairs. "Okay, get your balance. Careful, careful. Now head to the stairs. One foot at a time. Excellent, excellent. Another foot. Yes, excellent. Now straight ahead to the chair."

Some mornings I want to scream. Other mornings I drift through this routine with a measure of tranquility, moving without thinking too much, my mind looking ahead to the hour when Martha will arrive. Or I'll try to practice a little Zen, concentrating on just what I am doing, hoping to live precisely in the present. I'm still not very good at this.

Many years ago, when James and I vacationed on the northern California coast, I became friendly with the young woman who ran our bed-and-breakfast. Mimi described her sometimes difficult clients, the witless damage, the constant cleaning, the breakfasts that had to be prepared right on time, the multitude of chores. A devoted Zen disciple, Mimi told me, "My biggest test is when I'm cleaning a toilet. I turn the task into a meditation. I pay attention to my work, every gesture, every moment."

I wish for a touch of Mimi in the morning. Rather than savor the moment, I often feel as if time has alarmingly telescoped. I have just finished clearing up after breakfast, and now I need to get James into his pajamas. Where did the day go? How did I disappear? Why am I on this frozen tundra?

HOW IS JAMES?

April 13

"How is James?"

I struggle with an answer to this simple question. If James had a cold or flu or even pneumonia, I would know what to say. "Much better, thank you," or "His cold has turned quite nasty, but our doctor just put him on antibiotics, and he should be fine in a week or two." If he were recovering from a broken bone, I might still be able to produce a truthfully optimistic response.

But James has a chronic, progressive disease, and his Parkinson's never gets better. It only gets worse. Some Parkinson's patients do find symptomatic relief from new medications, brain stimulation, or other treatments. The disease, however, continues on its relentless downward path, and it never stops. An interviewer once asked former Supreme Court Justice Sandra Day O'Connor about her husband, who was then institutionalized with Alzheimer's. Her answer was succinct: "There is no good news with Alzheimer's." So it is with Parkinson's.

As I fumble for words, I remind myself that people ask me this question out of polite, kind, and sometimes loving motives. One motive is, understandably, the furtive curiosity with which we watch someone else face a decline toward death. Although we—the temporarily healthy ones—may pretend we can avoid this path, we still want to know how someone else walks it. What is happening now? What happens next? What is the end game? How will he play it? (How will we?)

Others, I sense, ask with a tinge of guilt. They are old friends of James's who do not call or visit because they cannot handle what has happened to the man they used to know. For these friends, I repress my own question that would make them truly uncomfortable: Why don't you drop by sometime and see for yourself?

How is James? Parkinson's is such a complicated disease, affecting every sufferer so differently. Over the years, I have had to ask many friends about someone's cancer. The answer—not the disease—can sometimes be straightforward: "He gets really sick from the chemo/radiation, and he is depressed" (or, sometimes, "keeping his spirits up"). If I had to describe only James's physical symptoms, I could be straightforward too: "Still walking, with a cane or walker." If anyone wanted to know more, I could continue, "Well, he is definitely weaker and tires easily. The tremor isn't bad. Some trouble swallowing now, though." Then we could move on; the subject has been covered.

When I have to figure dementia into the answer, I begin to stumble. My words turn into a stutter, as I try to be brief, descriptive, and yet not melodramatic. (I'm not going to say, "Some days this breaks my heart.") I want to avoid the word "dementia" if possible; it terrifies my listener. So I mention confusion and some memory loss instead. I have been asked too often, "So does he still recognize you?" or "Does he know where he is?" Yes and yes.

I could talk for ten or fifteen minutes, circling around the subject. I could explain that he needs some help when we watch a fast-moving DVD, but he still enjoys a carefully chosen movie. He can listen to an engrossing nonfiction audiobook that doesn't rely on plot. Also, I could go on, James loves having an aide read to him from a half-finished memoir we once wrote together about his architectural career. It was never published, but now it serves an unexpected purpose, offering a gentle springboard into a shrinking pool of memories.

I could add that James occasionally wakes up frightened and disoriented. He has terrible nightmares, quite common with Parkinson's. He forgets quickly at times, so that I need to tell him again and again, "No, not today. Your son Frank is coming to see you tomorrow." This refrain would sound familiar to anyone who knew someone with Alzheimer's.

Should I try to illustrate the veering between connecting and disconnecting? Today, for example. When Frank took James for a walk, Frank mentioned afterward how many dogs they'd stopped and petted. For most of his life, James had a dog. (Now, for several reasons, we have cats.) After Frank left, I settled James on the sofa for a short rest. He held my hand and looked up at me earnestly. I could tell he was struggling to tell me something. "I wonder . . . I think maybe not . . . but perhaps," he began. I waited. "I wonder," James forged on with determination, "if we shouldn't get a dog!"

By this time, my audience of one or two would be longing to escape. And I wouldn't have finished, wanting to add nuance, hoping to brush in all gradations for a full and honest portrait. Some days are worse, some better. How is James doing? I don't always know myself.

I now give silent thanks to Martin, a friend who saw me in a grocery-store parking lot and asked, "How is James these days?" I began my usual stumbling reponse, thinking, "Oh, God, this is so difficult," when Martin abruptly broke into my speech. Martin does not waste anyone's time; I have always liked this about him. "Okay," he said, "just tell me: on a scale of one to ten?"

Martin had handed me a solution. "Right," I said with relief. This I could handle. "One to ten, with James at his best at ten? Well, physically, I'd say about five. He can still walk, but he has trouble with balance, and he doesn't have much energy." Martin nodded. "And mentally?" I went on. "Well, some days I'd give him a seven, but other days he zooms down to a three. He isn't ever at a ten anymore." Martin shook his head. "Too bad," he said. "Too bad." I agreed, and Martin drove on.

Now when they ask, "How is James?" I could give them one to ten on two different scales. Then I'd let their imaginations go to work. Although I would answer further questions, I might not have to. As I've already learned, "seven down to three" tends to stop those questions anyway.

PRIORITIES: BLUE JEANS

April 20

Yesterday I had a choice. At midmorning I unexpectedly found myself with an hour and a half more or less free. Martha could stay until lunchtime. An hour and a half!

I did not even think of consulting my long-term, increasingly lengthy, very-soon-I-need-to-do-this list. Although this list can be a frustrating reminder, it is also an entirely irrational assurance that once everything is written down, those tasks are already halfway done.

I wanted to leave the house to buy a pair of jeans. I wouldn't have to go far; a consignment shop down the block has racks of inexpensive jeans waiting for new owners. I didn't actually need a new (to me) pair of jeans, in the sense that my old jeans were not yet threadbare. But they had become baggy, faded, and grubby looking. I was depressed by these jeans.

Morally, I felt, I should accomplish something tangible in my hour and a half, not waste my time struggling in and out of dozens of pairs of jeans. Adding an "e" to "moral," however, I could think of this as "morale," and a caregiver certainly needs to pay attention to that. The consignment store was so close and temptingly cheap. My closet was already bright with a rainbow spectrum of T-shirts, and I don't need dress-up clothes anymore.

When scuttling around the house, I get discouraged if I glance in a mirror and see a drab, grayish woman glancing back at me. So when I get dressed in the morning, I go for color. Especially at my age, I like a bit of flash. I love gaudy earrings. I own several inexpensive, jaunty, wide-brimmed hats. Even heading outdoors for a walk, I want to feel spiffy. After all, I need to remember I still exist. I am not only a caregiver.

I love my new jeans. They are midnight blue, they will go with every red or pink or purple top I own, and they fit just right. I looked in the mirror when I got home, and I recognized myself.

SMILING UNDER WATER

May 1

Today I am thinking how hard it is to be a good Buddhist. I haven't previously aspired to this—my aspirations these days are quite low, perhaps cooking a tender pot roast or riding my bicycle up a moderate hill without puffing—but I recently decided to try to follow Thich Nhat Hanh's precepts to bring more peace into my life. In his book *Present Moment, Wonderful Moment,* he makes this transformation sound so simple. He divides the day into ordinary activities, such as waking up, getting out of bed, and walking. For each activity, he has created a four-line poem, or "gatha." I am supposed to learn and then recite, mindfully, every gatha at the appropriate time.

I haven't been able to get past the first poem yet. It is not difficult to understand. "Waking up this morning, I smile. / Twenty-four brand-new hours are before me. / I vow to live fully in each moment / and to look at all beings with eyes of compassion."

I can recite the last two lines without irony. I wish I could always concentrate on the moment. I want to live as a compassionate being. Even if I mostly fail, try again, and fail once more, I know I am meant to keep trying, like coming up for air.

But I am stuck on the first two lines. Take the early morning smile. I practiced this (when I remembered) last week, feeling rather foolish, but nonetheless hoping it might affect how I approached my day. I have to admit that my smile felt artificial, a temporary fix of cosmetic surgery. But this morning a smile was not possible. I couldn't even imagine a smile.

James and I had arrived yesterday for a weekend at our cottage in the woods. Because of a treacherously icy winter, I have not been able to bring him here since last fall. The change from his usual environment, even to this familiar one, may have distressed him. At 2:00 a.m., James rang his bell for me. He needed to use the toilet. Fine. I'm here to do that. Glad to help. That's my job. At 2:25, he rang again. He wanted a drink of water. Well, yeah. Okay. But at 2:45 a.m., 3:30 a.m., 3:45 a.m., 4:30 a.m., on and on until 8:00 a.m., he had increasingly less coherent reasons for calling or ringing his bell. Sometimes he had no reasons at all. Unpredictable Parkie can play havoc with his mind at night.

It certainly plays havoc with mine. I'd bet most caregivers don't need a congressional investigation to know that having one's sleep constantly interrupted—finally falling back to sleep, only to be awoken once again, sinking back into the bed, jerking awake, again and again—is excruciating. One night is bad enough. Ten days of it, and I'd confess to anything.

When I gave up the fight for sleep at 8:00 a.m., helped James out of bed, and started to fix breakfast, I could barely bring myself to be civil. Poor James; it wasn't his fault. I was so tired that I was shaking. I was sinking again. Down, down, back under the water. Smile?

Now for the second line of the gatha: "Twenty-four brand-new hours are before me." Yes, I know. Life is very short, and as I age, my life is even shorter. I do not want to let those hours slip away. I want to pay attention to their possibilities.

But I soon learned what lay before me. Not long after breakfast, that day's aide, a sweet young woman from a nearby small town, arrived with the news she could only stay an hour. She had a last-minute job interview, an important one, and I agreed she had to go.

When James doesn't sleep at night, he does not make up his loss during the following day. He becomes jumpy, confused, even filled with nervous energy. He can sustain interest in a book, a CD, or any other amusement for only twenty minutes at a time. He wants to keep moving. On the second day, he is apt to take naps. But not on the first.

So I looked at those brand-new twenty-four hours and faltered. It was like looking down a familiar path I didn't want to follow. However, there it was. I took my first steps. I had no choice. And as I write this, the day has slowly moved along. We are getting through it. The sun has been shining off and on, and twice I have taken James outdoors for a short walk. At the moment he is listening to a recorded book about Britain in World War II; he has heard it before, but today I don't think he will notice. While he listens, I can write this.

In just four more hours, I will be getting James ready for bed again. Tonight he may sleep. Tomorrow morning I may resume practicing my smile. I might be smart to start practicing it under water.

BEIGE LIES, PINK LIES, PURPLE LIES

May 6

I am tired of lying. I've never had a problem giving deceptive answers to questions like, Is my new haircut flattering? Do you think I need to lose weight? or What did he really say about me? White lies are quick and easy.

I wish I didn't have to lie so much, and with such calculation, about caregiving. Last Saturday after breakfast, I repacked all the groceries, books, DVDs, and other essentials that were to have lasted for a long weekend at our cottage in the woods. Load after load, I trundled them back to the car in our wheelbarrow.

James had two terrible nights in a row, constantly waking and not knowing exactly what was happening. Nothing I could say or do soothed him back into sleep. Around 4:00 a.m. on the second night, I knew that in the morning I'd better get us home as soon as possible. If I had one more night like that, I knew I couldn't drive safely for two hours on high-speed roads.

As we headed out, I began wondering what I'd say to friends and family who knew how much I'd anticipated this spring weekend. They had heard about my longing to work in my untidy garden, to see violets and daffodils, to inspect the small reddish promise of peonies pushing into the light, to mulch my paths for the season. I don't have a garden in our small city lot.

Now I would have to answer their queries. "And did you have a fabulous weekend? What perfect weather! You must have been out in your garden all the time!"

This is what I'd really like to say about our weekend in the woods:

"Actually, it was a nightmare. James was unaccountably awake most of two nights, very disturbed, incoherent. My home aide disappeared. Since I couldn't leave James alone in the house, I wasn't able to get out to my garden at all.

"What I think troubled me more was knowing I might not be able to bring James here again. We have always loved this place so much. I wanted to burst into tears in the car, but I knew how that would upset him.

"As I drove, aiming the car steadily for home, I was a woman on a mission. Get us home. But I yearned for my garden. It keeps me rooted. These days my roots are frayed and drying, like a plant a squirrel had dug up and abandoned.

"We had endured such a hard winter. Saturday was so beautiful. But we had to leave."

If I had been truthful, I wouldn't have just said all this. I think I would have yelled it, like a small child wanting to rage and stamp her feet. I do sometimes pour out such honest reactions to a very few close friends. I always feel better afterward.

But to others, I consider my choice of lies.

Mostly I pick the beige lie. This is a white lie with a shading of truth, enough to add a slight off tinge that suggests not everything was completely wonderful. Beige lies are useful for people who are asking out of politeness. They really don't want details. They certainly don't want to hear a long wail of discouragement. But they have taken the trouble to ask, and I take a little trouble to answer.

So I might say about our aborted weekend at the cottage, "Oh, yes, the weather was great. James had trouble sleeping, so we came home early. Great weather, though. Lovely sunshine."

For those closer friends or family who deserve more truth but who would be distressed if I let them know how searing the weekend was, I'll produce a pink lie. A pink lie is darker than beige but adds a bit of rosiness at the end. So I'll give a fuller response but end with, "Maybe I can get there again before too long. I have to figure that out." (I don't know how I'm going to figure that out.)

Even when I'm almost telling the full truth, I often end up with a purple lie. A purple lie involves omissions that would saturate the truth, turning it into a dark, blood-red purple. These omissions are my darker thoughts, the ones I think many caregivers hear in their heads sometimes, like the rustle of bats in the night brushing against our faces. I am used to them now, and I let them flicker back and forth, trying to shoo them away before they can really sink their teeth into my spirit.

How, I wonder, could I explain, without alarming my listener, what I briefly thought the morning we left? Exhausted but driving with iron determination, I was carefully turning our car up a curving high hill. Tchaikovsky was soaring through the speakers, the sun was radiant, the green fields were flashing by. I was only driving the speed limit, 65 miles an hour, but I felt we were flying. "If we crashed right now," I thought for a moment, not actually wanting to crash, "this would be the way to go."

When I feel such dark thoughts pulsing below my cheerier words, I know I am telling someone a purple lie. Still, after I've recovered a little balance, I remind myself that in fact, when I talk about telling the truth, I only have an incomplete idea of what the truth is. My version changes, sometimes without my noticing, almost every day.

Today I can report that I drove this morning to a garden

center and brought home eight hanging plants. Hung on metal poles, they are lighting up our backyard: purple petunias, pale-pink double impatiens, and cherry-red geraniums. This is not my sprawling, extravagantly blowsy garden, but it helps. That, today, is the truth.

A VERY SHORT TOOTH TALE

May 7

I consulted my dentist yesterday. Two of my teeth, one upper and one just below it, seemed damaged. They hurt some of the time. When I drank or ate something cold, the upper tooth hurt even more. What was the problem?

I like my dentist, but I hate having any dental work. I even hate the sound of a polishing drill when I have my teeth cleaned. So I dreaded a diagnosis with words like "root canal," "abscess," or "infection."

My dentist tapped and poked. He blew cold air on the troubled spots (ouch!). He took an X-ray. He peered with his mirror and tapped some more.

"What we're seeing here," he finally concluded, "is caused by grinding or clenching your teeth."

He looked at me. I looked at him. He sees James too, and he knows what is happening.

"Oh, right," I said. I went home.

HANGING ON

May 25

During bad times—these last few weeks, for example, when James's dementia is noticeably worse and his hallucinatory nightmares ever more disruptive—I continue to be surprised by how a small gesture or unexpected comment can comfort me.

A few days ago, I did snag an overnight stay alone at our retreat in the Wisconsin woods. On the way home, I stopped at the Smiling Pelican bakery.

Sandra and David open this small-town, tiny, and wildly successful bakery only during the summer season. Sandra is a world-class baker who trained abroad. David, an artist, tends the counter. He is a man of very few words, polite but crisp. He does not invite personal conversation. But for years, as James and I stood in line for our chance at chocolate-bourbon truffles or pecan-pumpkin pie, I have asked a few questions. Unasked, I have volunteered information. So we have learned a little about each other.

This time I was alone. I had not seen David and Sandra since last fall. David said hello and waited for my order. I gave it to him. As he reached for a paper sack, he then asked, "How is James doing?" He had noticed James's absence.

I did not know whether David actually cared or not. But I was too tired for a lie. "Not very well," I said. I waited a moment. "I'm sorry I can't be more cheerful than that. But we are hanging on."

David put my sack on the counter. He looked directly at me. A moment passed. "Sometimes," he said slowly, "that's all we can do."

"Yes," I said.

In the car, I took a large bite from my chocolate-covered macaroon and continued driving home.

ABSENT FRIENDS

June 7

J ames and I are not used to being invisible.

Before Parkinson's bit so unshakably into James, and before I stopped writing in order to care for him, the two of us were certainly not celebrities, but we were not an unknown couple. Publicity about his architecture and my books appeared here and there.

During those active years, we were frequently invited to dinners and parties. James in particular brought amiability and energy to any gathering, and he reveled in telling anecdotes. Because I have always been curious about people, I like to ask questions, and I can tell a few stories too. So we found ourselves on some guest lists.

This was good news for James. He loved going out and entertaining in return, but I was much less eager for a social life. I was happier to stay at home with James. My idea of a blissful evening? A quiet dinner, a good book, PBS's *Mystery Theater*. This was one of the ongoing compromises in our marriage. We would both laugh when someone asked, "So, do you entertain quite a bit?" because James would always reply, "Oh, almost never!" and I would simultaneously groan, "Oh, yes, far too often!"

I thought of all this last week at a neighborhood barbeque.

The much younger and very nice couple next door, with two charming children, were the hosts. Together with other families in the block, they had planned a potluck, and they cordially invited us—even assuring me, kindly, that I would not need to bring anything. They do see the daily march of my caregiving aides coming and going.

All Sunday afternoon James was very excited. He kept asking if it was time to go to the party yet. (It wasn't.) His days are very much the same, so this barbeque sounded to him like a celebratory event. He hadn't been to a party for at least two or three years. We are no longer invited anywhere. This is not puzzling. James's difficulty in communicating makes conversation awkward. Poignantly, he still assumes that he would always be a welcome guest.

In late afternoon, when I heard voices and knew the party had begun, I told James—who was dressed very smartly for the occasion, bright sport shirt, colorful slacks—that we would go now but not remain long. "You need to eat by 6:00," I reminded him, "if we're going to get you to bed by 7:30. And I don't think we can stay for the barbeque itself."

"Oh, no," said James firmly, "I *want* to stay for the barbeque!"

"Well, we'll see," I said, but I dialed our oven to 350 degrees so I could pop two frozen salmon cakes inside as soon as we got home.

We crossed through a gap in the hedge to our neighbors' backyard. Several tables and chairs dotted the grass, and a table with drinks and snacks had been set up near the barbeque. Beyond the table, maybe four or five yards away, a cluster of ten or twelve people stood talking, clinking glasses, and laughing. We knew only a few of them.

Our neighborhood is a small enclave of mostly older, substantial houses, well kept up, close to a beautiful city lake. Many are newer homeowners, doctors, lawyers, or successful businessmen. They lead very active lives. Those we know always greet us cordially, but we seldom see them. We also no longer swim in forward-rushing currents.

James stood, leaning on his cane. "Shall we sit down?" I asked him, pointing to the nearest table.

"No, no, I want to stand!" he said impatiently. He kept looking eagerly toward the tight-knit group. I knew he wanted to join them. He always headed for the middle of any group of people who were enjoying themselves. But I didn't feel like edging forward, breaking into the fast chatter, and determinedly introducing ourselves. I also knew that, even if I did, James would not be able to enter into the conversation. I am not shy, but I was tired. Suddenly this all seemed too much effort.

For several minutes we stood by ourselves. Then I asked gently, "Shall we sit down now, James?" He nodded. We sat. Our hostess came over, greeted us graciously, and offered to fetch us drinks. Then she and I talked politely, until soon one of her children tugged at her arm. She moved away. Our thoughtful host also stopped by our table to welcome us.

After James had sipped his lemonade, and I had emptied my wine glass rather too quickly, he looked at the party going on before us. Several children were romping across the wide lawn, chasing each other and scrambling on the elaborate play equipment. The sun was shining, the grass was a luminous green, a breeze ruffled women's skirts. "Isn't this a wonderful scene?" he said. I agreed. He waited a few minutes and then repeated this remark. I agreed again. And it was: our neighbors and their children might have been in a commercial for Advil, Claritin, Lexapro, or any product that effortlessly smoothed out difficulties in life. White clouds, soothing and dreamy, drifted above us.

We stayed sitting at our table for half an hour. One of the guests we knew, Elsa, a recent divorcée, paused long enough to sit down and then tell us how hectic her weekend had been, lunch with a new escort, a dinner date with someone else, a night at the theater with friends. She was exuberant and happy. We told her we were very pleased for her. She moved on.

James finally turned to me and said, "I'm ready to go when you are." I helped him up, and as we passed our host at the barbeque grill, we thanked him. Elsa saw us leaving and waved good-bye.

As soon as we got inside our house, I put the salmon cakes into the oven and set the table. Before long, James and I were eating our supper. I was relieved to be home. Then, as I was clearing away the dessert plates, he looked out the window toward our neighbors and said, "I felt so bad." He paused. "I felt so bad."

I sat down next to him again. "At the party?" I asked, knowing the answer.

"Yes," he said. "I couldn't . . . I couldn't . . ." He was unable to finish his sentence; this often happens. He looked so sad. "I just couldn't . . . like I wanted."

"I know," I told him, patting his hand gently. "You couldn't participate the way you used to." He nodded. "It's this rotten Parkinson's," I said. "It's not your fault."

James looked away from the window and straight at me. "I didn't know I would feel this bad," he said. Parkinson's tends to mask facial expressions, but James's eyes and the quiver of his mouth were eloquent.

"Listen, James," I replied. I am sure I sounded fierce. "I want to tell you something. I love our location. I love this house. We've lived here a long time, but people around here are very . . ." I looked for the right words, stumbling a little. "They are very locked into their own lives. And"—here I thumped the table for emphasis—"we are *not* going to any more neighborhood parties. *Not, not, not!* Now let's find that Adam Dalgliesh DVD and watch a little before you have to go to bed."

James cheered up, we sat on the sofa together in front of the TV screen, and he did not mention the party again.

Later that night, after James was asleep, I sat up for an hour to read before going to bed myself. I thought about the party. So this is what it feels like to be disabled and ignored. If I had been in that laughing, chatting group, would I have made the necessary effort? Would I have walked over to greet an older couple sitting alone together? I liked to think so, but was I sure?

When I thought how much James missed the social interaction that was once such a vital part of his life, I wanted to weep. I dismissed from my mind the neighbors we barely knew. But I wondered, not for the first time, about so many of James's old friends who had gone missing. During his long career, he had mentored, nurtured, and rejoiced in the companionship of many of his former students. In turn, many of them kept in contact, phoning James for lunch (and advice), telling him over and over how much he had meant to them over the years. He was always touched by this attention.

In former days, when we went out to lunch together, one or more people almost always came over to our table to greet James. Other stopped us on the street. Our city is large, but in his circle, James was well known and much respected. I always noticed the number of men and women who spoke to him with such affection.

They are gone now. In the early years of his Parkinson's, when James was still so much his old self, he used to go out to lunch almost every day. He savored those genial occasions, full of camaraderie and gossip, usually enhanced with a glass of white wine. He drove then, and his favorite restaurant was downtown, near his old office, so he could also stop in to check what was happening there. He relished those visits too. Almost every weekday morning he called someone, maybe a friend of forty years, or a high school classmate he saw only twice a year, or a former student who was temporarily out of work and needed cheering up. Many calls came to our house too. James was still in demand.

As his Parkinson's slowly worsened, we adjusted. I sometimes made those calls for him. When he stopped driving, I arranged taxis, and sometimes our aide Martha dropped him off, did errands or took a walk, and then picked him up to take him home.

Then after a time, except for his grown children calling, the phone seldom rang for James. He found it harder to engage in back-and-forth conversation. His speech was often halting, his memory patchy. Whoever lunched with him needed to settle James in his chair, to help with the menu, to wait patiently as he found the right words. Although James no longer could regale anyone with his long, complicated jokes, and he had fewer stories to tell, he listened with attentive eagerness to his companions. He came home from his lunches with a visible glow. But the lunches were now very rare.

Pondering what I could do, I asked for advice from Mick, a younger friend whom he had once encouraged and sustained during a prolonged personal crisis. "What you need to do," Mick told me, "is set up a shared caring circle. I've been a member of one myself. You simply organize a few of James's friends who really care about him, and you ask them to meet at your house from time to time to talk about what James needs. Then they help provide it. Trust me: a caring circle is a fantastic experience for everyone concerned."

I couldn't quite picture myself presiding at our dining-room table (where would James be?) during these meetings. But I tossed the caring circle idea around in my mind, and I finally decided to try a less demanding version of it. I sent a joint e-mail to three of James's longtime friends, all of whom James had greatly helped, with pleasure, at the start of their careers. I stressed that I was writing because James had such a special relationship with each of them. I explained in my e-mail how much James enjoyed his time with them.

I noted I knew that having lunch with James wasn't as easy as it once had been. "If you could separately find time in your very busy lives to see him every six weeks or two months, that would make him very happy," I wrote. "I can arrange transport. Or you could visit him here. It doesn't have to be a long visit."

I did know their lives were very busy. Everyone has a very busy life. But surely, I thought, this heartfelt appeal would crack open a door that was slowly but steadily shutting in James's open, eager face.

The door did not budge. The wife of one of my chosen three called me and suggested setting up a lunch for the four of us. It turned out that she wanted me to talk to her church group. A second did call, many weeks later, and said he was about to leave for England and Scotland but would get in touch when he returned. He wondered if I could suggest some places to stay in London. We talked for quite a while about his trip, and I spent an hour on the Internet to find the right suggestions. He was very appreciative. But he never did call after his return. The third arranged one lunch, but—"This was great! We'll have to do it again soon!"—he did not try again.

For decades, James had attended a congenial, radically liberal Catholic church. Two other members of this church—one was Mick, the other Bart—often joined James for coffee and croissants afterward. They discussed the sermon, the church, the state of the world. When James could no longer get up early enough for the service, he asked me to call Bart and urge him to come over for a visit. "Oh, yes, I'll do that really soon," Bart said firmly. "You know what? I could come and read to him. I'd be happy to do that. Of course I'll come." Weeks passed. Could I call Bart again, James wondered? This time I left a message on Bart's answering machine. Bart never returned my call.

Another friend, Glenn, a literally high-flying entrepreneur, who used to stop by every few weeks, took to phoning from the airport, just as he was about to depart for Chicago, San Francisco, or New York. I think he was filled with good intentions as he sat, bored, with cell phone in hand, at the departure gate. "Give my best to James," he'd say, and then add, "Tell him that as soon as I get back, we'll have to get together." I felt like interrupting and bursting into an old lyric that James used to sing with off-key mischievousness: "It seems to me I've heard that song before / It's from an old familiar score / I know it well, that melody." That was James's way of saying, "Oh, yeah, like that's ever going to happen!"

Not everyone has deserted. One of his oldest friends, Dan, who now spends five months every winter in the temperate Southwest, sends James a short note or clipping or card once or twice every week that he is gone. James loves getting those greetings. He doesn't focus on what Dan writes as much as on the fact that Dan has remembered him. "Oh, look!" I cry, bringing in the mail. "A card from Dan!" James smiles broadly and reaches for it. I prop each one up on the dining table until another arrives.

Eben, our beloved doctor, and Sean, partners in a whirlwind of work, volunteer activities, an active spiritual group, gardening, bicycling, and much more, call us every week. Eben regularly brings over a large pan of his delectable lasagna, and we once lived happily for several days on a huge pot of Sean's split-pea soup. Watching James's decline, they continue to make sure he feels fully included in any of our quiet suppers together. After they have left, sometimes James's eyes fill with tears of gratitude for their friendship.

A much younger man, Steven, one of James's last protégés, to whom James had become quite close, somehow finds space, despite the demands of a rapidly rising career and an active family life, to call or visit often enough so that James never feels forgotten. Even as James's dementia and confusion worsens, he will almost leap to his feet and call out "Steven!" with great happiness as his young friend enters the room. Although James often laments to me afterward, "I couldn't contribute much," that has not yet deterred Steven.

On long afternoons, when I know James would so much enjoy company, I sometimes indulge myself in composing a little speech. I imagine myself delivering it at James's funeral. (Widows do not usually give speeches. This one probably will.) I wouldn't want to be vengeful, I tell myself. No, no, certainly not.

Maybe I could say something like this: "I want to thank those of you who interrupted your very hectic lives to spend a little time with James in these last months and years. He valued your visits more than you'll ever know. Your kindness meant a great deal to both of us, and I hope someday, if you are old and infirm, you will find that attention repaid in turn to you." Then I picture myself smiling one of my phoniest smiles and running a piercing laser beam over the crowd. I look for Bart, Glenn, and some others. I silently dare them to come up to me at the reception and express their sympathies.

No, caregiving has not made me a saint.

This nastier turn of mind does fade. I try not to stay angry; James would not approve. Besides, I think I know what has happened. Some people simply cannot bear to see James in a diminished state, his former lighthearted banter reduced to stumbling speech, his quick intelligence dulled. They want to remember him as he was before Parkinson's. When they see James now, perhaps they also see themselves, some years in the future. Maybe for them that future looks closer and closer. Americans tend to warehouse our elders—if not literally shoving them out onto the ice, then moving them conveniently out of sight. Once there, we let someone else take responsibility. Someone else can talk to them. Someone else can bend close, listen carefully, and try to decipher what needs to be said or done. So few of us spend much time with the old, especially with the demented.

The very word "dementia" scares away people. Talking about James to his friends, I try to use other phrases: "often confused," "difficulty in communicating," "short-term memory loss." "Dementia," translated from my foggy Latin, suggests that someone is "out of (the) mind"—when in fact his dementia can be fluid, partial, a cloud that moves and darkens but then drifts for a while, letting sunshine through in redeeming shafts of light.

I can understand why it is terrifying. We are all afraid of losing our minds—or being thrown "out of the mind" into some dizzying perplexity or baffling darkness. Yet many people do visit terminally ill patients with cancer, liver disease, congestive heart failure. When James is still softly radiating—though in a much muted way—his zest for life, why do those friends stay away?

I will never know, because they will never tell me. Not long ago, Ray, now in his sixties, who as a young student was so close to James and his family that they considered him almost a son and brother, called me from his office in Denver. He makes this call every few months. "So how is James?" he asks. After I've answered his question—vaguely, if James is listening—I hand the phone to James. "Well, Raymondo!" James almost booms this nickname into the telephone, his often faint voice now animated with pleasure. To him, Ray will always be the smart, irreverent young man he loves.

What I don't understand is why Ray has not seen James in a decade. He has an aging parent in this city, whom he occasionally visits. These visits have gone on for years. But we don't know when Ray comes and goes. He never calls us when he is in town. After his last phone inquiry, which I answered in a room where James couldn't hear, I said, "Ray, if you ever want to have a real conversation with James in person, now is the time. Or it won't happen."

Then I felt an arrow loose itself from a quiver I didn't know I was holding. "I just want to say one other thing, Ray," I heard my voice let fly. "If you don't come to see James before he dies, don't bother to come to the funeral. I'm not kidding. Just don't bother."

"Gotcha," said Ray. "I hear what you're saying."

"Okay, now I'll get James on the phone. He'll be so glad to talk to you," I said. I knew that distant, bodiless connection was all James was going to get. I was sorry—for Ray as well as James—and for all the absent friends who do not know what they have really lost.

NO SKIPPING TO THE LAST PAGE

June 23

> *This alarm bell rang more than a year before James actually died. Parkinson's defies prognosis.*

"So how does it end? Does anyone really important die?" I ask my daughter, who has just recommended a movie. I have read a few reviews; the critics haven't given much away.

"Oh, Mom, you don't want me to tell you!" Jenny wails. She shouldn't have to wait for my answer. She's had this conversation with me many times.

"I just want to know if it ends happily," I say firmly. These days I have no intention of going to a movie that will leave me depressed. I don't even want to see a movie that is sad but uplifting. Uplifting, okay. Just not sad.

"Okay, okay," she groans. "I can't believe you really want to know. But yes, it does. Mostly."

"Mostly? How mostly?" I press her.

"Oh, come on, Mom," she says with some irritation. "Nothing you can't handle. Really."

"Good," I say. "Then I'll try to see it."

I am uneasy about endings. As an avid reader, sometimes I become so involved in a novel that I begin to worry too much about what will happen to the characters—a pair of lovers, a lonely child, an agonized mother. I dread coming to the final chapter only to discover a terrible loss or a permanent parting. Slogging through *Cold Mountain* several years ago, I almost threw the book down afterward, feeling I'd been suckered. After hundreds of pages, he gets *killed?*

So I cheat. Although I am a little embarrassed to admit this, I have been known—James has caught me at this—to peek for a few moments, just skimming, at the last few lines or paragraphs of a book. Then, my anxieties relieved, I can return to the story and continue, letting the complications unfold, onward to the conclusion. Or I may decide to just flutter the pages and catch the highlights. After all, if that is how it is going to end . . .

I am thinking about endings right now. A few days ago, James and I consulted with Dr. Janet Sutton, our Parkinson's specialist. Or perhaps I should say that I consulted. James was there, listening, speaking haltingly, but I was the one asking questions. In the past six weeks, James's disease seems to have taken another huge bite. He has developed recurrent sleeplessness that may or may not be sundowner syndrome, a lighthearted phrase for a very disturbing condition in which someone suffering from mental confusion takes a sharp turn for the worse as the afternoon wanes into evening. Medications of all sorts have not really helped. He is also less alert. I catch fewer moments of sparkle in his eyes. He continues slowly to lose weight.

As I explained James's symptoms, Janet listened carefully. She is an expert in this disease. She has seen James as a patient for many years. When Janet speaks—and she never blathers or fudges—I pay attention. Then Janet leaned back in her chair, and she said, choosing her words carefully, with compassion but utter clarity, "I consider that it is part of my job to tell patients and their families when I think I see an end approaching. James does not fit the usual pattern. I tend to watch for a situation when someone can no longer walk or talk or when someone loses weight rapidly. That is not happening here. But I do think that you are probably entering the final chapter."

Janet went on to explain, again with great care, that with Parkinson's, a "final chapter" might be months. It might be a year, even two years. Or, she added, change might come very rapidly.

Only two weeks ago, James had a physical exam with our family doctor. All its results were fine. I mentioned this to Janet. "Yes," she said, with a rueful smile at James, "below the neck, you seem to be in excellent shape. But you do have a progressive neurological disease, and it is getting worse." She paused for a moment and looked at me. "I do think that this is the time to get in touch with family members and tell them if anything remains to be said, they should say it now. If anyone has unfinished business, this is the time to take care of it." I nodded.

During her short summation, James had his head down. I wasn't sure he was grasping what she was saying. But when I gently tilted his head up, I could see tears in his eyes. "Do you understand what Janet is telling us?" I asked him. He finds it hard to utter complete sentences, but he looked at me, and I could hear the catch in his voice when he said, "Of course I understand. How could I not understand?"

I talked then for a short while, partly for Janet but mostly for James, not for the first time, about the incredible richness that has filled his life, our happy twenty-eight years together, our love for each other, and my nondoctrinal belief in the continuing power of love. I had tears in my voice too. I held his hand very tightly.

We did not stay much longer. When Janet asked James if he had any questions or something else on his mind, he waited a little. I could tell he was searching for words. "I'm just glad," he said, stopping often to gather this thought, "that I have someone pleasant to be with." "Pleasant" may not have been the exact word he wanted, but I knew what he meant. I smiled a little and asked,

"Do you mean me or Janet?" We still can sometimes tease each other.

As we left, Janet put her hand on my shoulder. "You know how to get in touch with me," she said quietly.

On the way home, James was silent. This was not remarkable. He doesn't talk easily anymore, and he has great powers of denial. He also forgets quickly. But when we drove by a city lake, far enough from our house that we have never strolled there together, he unexpectedly asked, "Can we take a walk?"

It was a very hot, sunny, summer afternoon, and I had a headache. I had not brought my sunhat or his walker. Of course I stopped the car anyway, and we very slowly walked a short distance along the path by the shore. I clutched his arm with all my strength, and he used his cane. We did not talk, but we held onto each other. Then we got back into the car and went home.

Now I cannot stop thinking about endings. This rather surprises me. After all, nothing Dr. Sutton said was news to me. I've known that James has had Parkinson's for many years; I am aware he is eighty-four; I have seen him slowly fade these past months. But the end of the last chapter seems so much closer. It is pressing against my shoulder; it is waving a warning hand before my face.

A few days after we had visited Dr. Sutton, I arranged to have morning coffee with a new friend who has become a wonderful confidante and comfort. Barb leads a crowded professional life. We do not see each other often. But Barb has measured out my path, and she knows the cost of each agonizing step. When we meet, she always opens her arms, and I usually start to cry.

On this morning, we talked about what Janet had told James and me. Barb walked me back through her own last months with her much-loved husband. We also spoke about grief, before and afterward, and the tenuous possibility of a future. Sometimes I could glimpse a pinpoint of light flickering in my own darkness. Frequently I glanced at my watch. I had to be back at my house in an hour.

Just before we hugged and parted, Barb said, "One thing I can tell you. The day will come when you are no longer automatically looking at your watch every fifteen minutes."

I knew exactly what she meant. I have time now. I do not want to let it slip through my fingers unnoticed. I want to use it well. But I do not want to think about time constantly either. And I cannot bear to skip ahead to the last page.

MY ADVENTURES WITH GENTLEMEN'S PADS

July 5

Life goes on, except when it doesn't. So despite James's and my official launch into the last chapter, I continue with everyday details of caregiving.

I try not to look ahead. Sometimes, however, I look back. I only began writing these entries in February, yet February now seems so long ago, frozen in a distant past. In February James slept fairly well most nights, he could feed himself without much help, and I could plan an overnight break without wondering whether I'd be able to leave. That was February. Now is harder.

As I look back, I wonder what I've learned. I don't necessarily focus on the Big Topics: achieving patience, savoring the present moment, celebrating what is possible. My grasp of these virtues is often elusive.

What I do realize, often with wry amusement, is how I've accumulated extensive knowledge on subjects I could never have before imagined. "Gentlemen's pads," for instance. That's what I call them in our house. I don't use the phrase "adult diapers." When James and I began this journey together, I fervently wished I had a caregiving handbook as useful as Dr. Spock was for my generation of parents. I needed a reassuring compendium of facts with a comprehensive index. Instead I had to research and learn about gentlemen's pads myself.

When I opened a previously undiscovered door into the crowded world of home health aids, medical supplies, and incontinence care, I was amazed at its detail and complexity. I had my first glimpse of this world several years ago. As I told my friend Grace that I was about to undergo a routine first colonoscopy, she interrupted with great emphasis. "Susan, get yourself to a drugstore right away and buy an adult diaper. You'll want it for the night before and the next morning. I'm not kidding."

At my local Walgreen's, I had many times walked down the aisle where adult diapers were stacked without giving them a glance. This time I stopped, looked, and wondered how to make sense of the assorted large boxes with bright-colored lettering. Some products were labeled for men, but others seemed unisex. The only brand I recognized was Depends. That was because June Allyson, the sunny, pretty star of many of my favorite musicals in the 1950s, appeared years later in Depends ads. (I remember thinking sadly, "Has it come to this?" It had.)

After I'd lingered in the aisle for a while, I began to feel self-conscious. Other shoppers passed me, and although I am sure I only imagined they were staring at me curiously, I kept wanting to say, "I only need to buy one. Really! Just for tonight!" Finally, deciding Grace had probably been overcautious, I decided to leave Walgreen's with just a tube of toothpaste. (Too late, I learned Grace had given me excellent advice.)

So although I knew where to find adult diapers, I still knew nothing about them.

For the first seven years or so of James's Parkinson's, I didn't need to think about medical supplies. We made a few changes in our living arrangements—grab bars here and there, a chair with arms and rollers for easy access to the dining table, wooden handholds (cleverly engineered by his son) to fasten onto James's bed for help in getting up. For a long time, James was able to arise at night and walk a very few steps down a hall into the bathroom. Then he couldn't. His balance and coordination became uncertain.

Eventually I realized we should acquire a commode, something that could sit right next to James's bed, involving only a few steps. I knew nothing about commodes either.

After checking the Yellow Pages and Google, then making a few phone calls, I visited my first medical-supply store. It was only a small, cluttered annex inside a mini-mall drugstore, but it was quite an introduction to the ingenuity and variety of inventions to ease a life with disabilities. On my way to a room housing large items like walkers, wheelchairs, and commodes, I passed shelf after shelf of specially designed plates, flatware, glasses, long tongs for picking up dropped items, trays, bibs, bed rails, folding canes, pillows for knees or feet or necks, support braces, splints, disposable gloves, bed tables, doorknob grippers, elastic shoelaces, on and on. I was fascinated, the way I feel in a well-stocked hardware store, as I wandered among tools and devices I did not know existed and that now seemed essential. (I bought, in fact, a hip-length plastic-backed bib, in a cheerful tartan, with adjustable neck snaps. It has been very useful.)

Once I found myself among the array of commodes, I needed to summon help. What was a bariatric commode? (Answer: one designed for an especially heavy person.) Did I need one with drop arms? One that folded? With a backrest? Why did they all have to be hospital white with gleaming metal frames?

"Well," said the saleswoman, "I can show you one that isn't on the floor yet. It just came in." She paused and then added impressively, "It is the Cadillac of commodes."

A Cadillac? So were these others Chevies? She soon returned, lugging a blue chair. It did indeed look different. Its back and arms were upholstered in a bright blue padded plastic, as was the contoured seat with matching padded lid. The chair trim was enameled black. Like any commode, it had a removable pail, its cover hidden under the cushy seat.

As I studied this Cadillac of commodes, relieved that it didn't instantly evoke a hospital room, the saleswoman added encouragingly, "This is of course more expensive, but considering that it is dual purpose, I think it is quite a bargain." I looked blankly at her. "You can also use it as an extra dining-room chair," she explained. I had a moment's vision of a dinner guest plopping himself down on this commode with its padded cover and trying to pretend he didn't know what it was.

Of course I bought this commode. In our house, bright blue will always beat hospital white. Installing it took two visits from our genius-of-all-trades, Blair, who keeps our house (and me) from falling down. A commode, I soon discovered, slides dangerously on a polished wood floor. So Blair constructed small wooden squares with doughnut holes just the size of the commode's legs. He fastened the squares to our floor with small screws. The legs were now immobile. I thought all was well.

With a chronic disease, nothing works for very long. James began to fall into such a confounding sleep that he could not wake up in time to use the commode. He was not incontinent—an unpleasant word, I think, carrying with it an undeserved whiff of blame—but he needed help. He needed, in fact, something protective to wear at night. I needed more protective equipment, too. Damp sheets and pajamas can mean a lot of laundry; a damp mattress is much more serious.

Off I went to Walgreen's again. Clueless as I was (why did none of my high-minded caregiving manuals talk about this?), I ended up with products that turned out to be next to useless. After buying and bringing home several cartons of a particular brand chosen more or less at random, I found that the briefs were fastened by sticky tabs. That meant that once one was pulled off, it could not easily be refastened again. The whole brief would have to be junked. For someone who might get up several times in the night, that was a lot of expensive briefs.

"Keep them," advised Martha. "They can be very useful if someone becomes bedbound. Easy to change." So in one downstairs closet, where I used to stash our travel supplies, I now have a large quantity of pristine sticky-tab diapers, which I hope I never have to use.

Back to Walgreen's. I clearly needed a pull-up undergarment, something with an elastic waist. Small? Medium? Large? Measurements vary with manufacturer. The labels were misleadingly uninformative; every box promised it was "Extra-absorbent," "Maximum," "Superior Absorbency," "Overnight," "Super-plus." Nothing, it seemed, was merely "Standard" or "Regular." All were superlative. I bought a variety for testing.

Fortifying James's bed took further research. I had no problem searching online for a high-quality waterproof mattress cover, soft quilted cotton on one side, not hospital-style crackly plastic. A return to the now-familiar Walgreen's aisle provided me with boxes of disposable plastic-backed square pads, rather like cheap small tablecloths, that could sit on top of the bottom sheet. If wet, the pad simply got tossed into the garbage.

Neither James nor I liked these pads. They wrinkled easily, they slithered, and they sounded like tissue paper as he tossed and turned. Another aide, Sandy, took me aside for some advice. "What you need is a heavy pad with a soft cotton surface, waterproof on the lower side, that you launder and use again and again. Buy two or three of them."

On to Google. After typing in "incontinence products," I became a little dazed by all the sites Google proffered, each offering various sizes, materials, weights, and prices. But I soon selected several bed pads, and, as Sandy had predicted, they were just what I needed. They lay sturdily on top of the sheet, and if one was damp, I could whip it off and replace it instantly. Near James's bed I learned to keep a colorful open canvas cube with clean pajamas and another with spare pads and even a spare sheet and mattress pad, just in case. Before long I could effect the necessary change in minutes, with minimum fuss, before James had to fully wake up.

I was still not finished with my research. None of the

gentleman's pads seemed to fully do the job. I could understand why. As I examined them, they seemed remarkably flimsy, with padding that hardly seemed to warrant the claims of "Extra-absorbent" or "Overnight Plus." To my eye, they might deal with leakage, but they could hardly hold an excreted glass of water.

Back, once again, to Walgreen's. Aha! Here were "male guards," closely resembling the old-fashioned, thick and bulky sanitary napkins that my generation of women used to buy as Modess or Kotex Super. All I needed to do was apply a male guard inside a gentleman's pad, and James would have double the protection, right?

Wrong. The male guard didn't seem to guard very much at all. I still found myself dealing with major laundry, and poor James with discomfort.

Now I ran through the Yellow Pages. I talked to local drug-stores and medical-supply outlets. Helpful salespeople sent me samples. Nothing worked.

I began to troll through Google once more; Google becomes a good friend to caregivers. Several medical-supply companies in far-flung states offered various incontinence products and brands I hadn't encountered in my safaris through Walgreen's. Every company also had a customer service department, and these sales-people, when I located them, always offered to send me samples. (All were discreetly delivered in brown paper packages with no identifying markers, as if I'd ordered pornography.) But none of the vaunted gentleman's pads ("This is our finest product!" "I'm sure you'll find this will solve the problem!") seemed much better than what I'd already tried.

These conversations with Incontinence Specialists—that was a title one company proudly used—were often memorable. My favorite was a long talk I had with a lady in a Deep South state. Her gentle, soothing drawl immediately made her sound like an intimate friend. Dolly (I'll call her) asked me several questions about James's needs. Then, pondering what to suggest, she asked me, in a circumlocution that took several minutes for me to figure out, "Well, dear, I need to know something important. Does your husband sleep on his back?" Yes, I assured her, always. He could not turn in bed anymore.

"Ah," she said. Silence. "So, umm, does his, well, his, um, well, you know, his, um, well, his masculine part. His, you know, member . . ." She was fumbling for words. "You mean," I said, hoping I wasn't sounding too crude to this refined lady, "his penis?"

"Yes, when resting . . . does it, would you say, always fold over to the right or to the left? That can make a difference, you know."

Now it was my turn for silence. I was embarrassed, not by her question—though later I wondered exactly why it made a difference—but by the fact that, alas, I didn't have an answer. James and I had enjoyed a happy marital relationship (as Dolly would doubtless have put it), but evidently I had just failed an important test of intimacy.

"I'm afraid I don't know," I told Dolly. She asked me a few more questions, and when I mentioned male guards, she said, "Oh, my. I think I've solved your difficulty. Those kinds of products have a waterproof backing. So when you put a male guard into a diaper, the, um, liquid can't flow into the padding of the diaper. Instead it just spills over the sides." This made sense. Dolly recommended a booster pad, which had no such backing, and therefore would provide the added absorbency I was seeking. Dolly was right.

When I think of my adventures with gentlemen's pads, I remember, still with some humiliation, what happened next. A few days after my discussion with Dolly, I e-mailed an old but faraway friend, Leslie, who during James's recent decline has sent me almost daily lively missives. Before her marriage, Leslie—a very attractive woman—had enjoyed many, many experiences with men Dolly would probably describe as "gentleman callers." They called, and they often stayed. Leslie knew all about what Dolly would call "very personal information."

"Listen, Leslie," I wrote her. "I want to ask you about something weird." I recounted my conversation with Dolly regarding the resting position of James's, um, masculine member. Was I remiss? Should I have known this? Is it indeed an important fact?

"Oh, yes," Leslie wrote back the next day. "She was quite right. Really, everybody knows that. A tailor always asks a man about it when measuring for a custom-made suit."

Everybody knows that? Oh. I decided not to discover what alteration, considering left or right, the tailor might then need to make in a pair of trousers. A loosish bulge? A discreet bit of extra fabric? A tad of backing? No, I let the subject lapse. Concluding my foray into the world of gentleman's pads, I thought, it was fitting to end with a reminder of my ignorance. I already knew more than I wished I'd ever had to learn.

THE VOICE IN THE
BATHROOM CUPBOARD

August 19

When I heard the voice, I was brushing James's teeth. I was already cloaked in the murky fog that envelops me around 5:00 p.m. By that time, my caregiving help has left for the day. I was facing a nonstop haul toward James's bedtime.

As I was dabbing with Kleenex to keep toothpaste off the floor, I suddenly heard a sharp, clear voice. It seemed to come from the bathroom cupboard behind me. "THIS WILL NEVER END," it said, in an authoritative tone. I kept brushing, but the voice didn't stop. "IT WILL NEVER END. IT WILL GO ON FOREVER. FOREVER." The voice seemed to fill the room. I knew whose voice that was. It was mine.

Two days ago, we went for James's two-month checkup with his Parkie specialist. Two months ago, we sat in Dr. Sutton's office as she told us, gently but firmly, that we were in the final chapter. We talked about endings. One of James's children had urged me to ask Dr. Sutton at our next visit about whether James was eligible for hospice care. So I did.

"No," Janet said, without hesitation. "I think hospice is a wonderful resource, and I will definitely let you know when I think that time has come. But James is still walking and talking."

(I thought to myself: actually, not so much talking. Or walking, either.) "I watch for certain markers. But in the absence of serious weight loss, or other severe changes, Parkinson's can go on for a very long time. Oh, no, it is not yet time for hospice. You have many, many steps downward still to come."

For the past two months, I had been thinking like an inexperienced marathon runner. (I'm not sure; I've never run a marathon.) Fifteen miles to go? Whew. I'm not sure I can do it. But maybe, trying to pace myself, I can last for at least five miles. Then I get to the five-mile marker, and I think, "Okay. I'm almost flattened, but maybe I can stagger another mile or two." At seven miles, I get a second wind. But at ten miles, I think I'm done. All in. No more energy. Knees wobbly. Breathing in gasps. And yet I keep going. Finally, I think I see the end marker. I know it is still far ahead, but it is almost visible. And as I approach, the marker vanishes. A new one appears. This one reads: "Forty miles. Keep running."

I have only a few close friends with whom I share this voice. It sounds so cold-blooded. I love James more than I could have ever thought possible. I still cannot picture a life without him.

Yet I can't get this voice, implacably issuing its stern sentence, out of my head. So now one of those trusted friends, whose own husband died a year ago after a prolonged decline, often sends me an e-mail in a hallucinatory, colored typeface. It is the same message. Between funky brackets that say "FLASH! FLASH!" are the words "IT WILL END! IT WILL END!"

I've told her to keep those flashes coming.

JUST A MINUTE!

September 3

Because James and I are somewhere—no one knows exactly where—in the final chapter, I'd like to think that the words he hears from me most often now are "I love you."

Actually, what he hears most often is *just a minute!* I say that phrase, calmly or irritably, reassuringly or dramatically, even sometimes with a screech, so many times a day that I should have a wristband recorder that would shout it out cheerfully when I press a button. I have many variations of tone for *just a minute!* Cheerful isn't always one of them.

James deserves a cheerful voice. Since I do not constantly hover over him, he sometimes has to call for me if he needs something. He may be feeling "discombobulated," his word for panicky confusion. Maybe he is chilled. Perhaps, bored with a DVD, he is anxious to get up from his chair. (Because he can so easily stumble, I have to use a red-corded ribbon tied loosely around him, reminding him to ask for help before rising.) He could simply be wondering where I am.

When he calls for me (and I'm never very far away), I am always doing something. I may be on telephone hold with the furnace repairman. I could be sorting through the mail. I may have just answered the doorbell. I'm feeding the cats, emptying the washing machine, holding the garbage sack in my hand as I head to the back door to deposit it in the trash can. I'm fixing supper. I'm washing the cooking pots. I'm putting away dishes.

Whatever I'm doing, I need a few seconds, maybe even a few minutes, before I drop the garbage or hang up the phone. Sometimes I can't quite understand what he wants; his voice is faint from Parkinson's. If I'm unsure, I do hurriedly drop the garbage. It could be an urgent cry for help.

If I'm focused on something, whether breading a piece of fish or unscrewing a stuck jar lid or sneaking a quick glance at Maureen Dowd's column in that day's paper, I am startled by his call. It breaks into my concentration like a fire alarm: "Susan! Susan!" Before I can help myself, I say, either under my breath or petulantly—depending on whether James can hear me— "[BLEEP!]," and then I yell, "Just a minute!" Sometimes I repeat myself, in a frustrated bleat: "Just a minute, James! Just a minute! *Just . . . a . . . minute!*"

After all this time as a caregiver, I still can't get used to this sense of constant pending interruption. Until James goes to bed, I exist in a state of fragmentation.

When my older sister was here on a recent visit, she felt I needed to relax more. She persuaded me to order a nifty biofeedback device, small enough to fit into my palm, with a video screen that measures breathing patterns. With little triangles and soft beeps, it tells me when to exhale. Then, after I end my session, it informs me how many "points" of relaxed breathing I've achieved.

I quite like this little device. I am proud of myself when I've achieved thirty-five or fifty points in ten or twenty minutes. According to the handbook of instructions about how to transform my life, relaxing here, relaxing there, I should be doing this several times a day—and definitely logging in one hundred points at bedtime. Then, in a few months, my instructions say, I will be quite a different person.

The problem is that I can't count on ten or twenty uninterrupted minutes. When I sink into a chair—James is napping on the nearby sofa—after a few minutes of breathing in . . . 1, 2, 3, 4 . . . (beep!) . . . breathing out . . . 1, 2, 3, 4 . . . I hear a rustling noise. James's shoes are squeaking on the leather cushion. Then he sits up. I open my eyes. He looks at me. "*What?*" I say, not in a very nice way. I turn my little device off.

If only I could float peacefully on the debris of the day, then I wouldn't feel so jangled by interruptions. Don't concentrate; don't get involved; don't open a book or read an e-mail. Like many people, I have become something of an e-mail addict. Unable to get out for more than a smidgen of social life, I rely on e-mails from near and far.

When James needs to use the bathroom, I tell him, "Call me when you're done," and close the door. I could sit on the nearby staircase and look at the wall. But I am only a few steps from my study. My computer is on the desk. Its screen glows. So I sit down.

Sometimes James is in the bathroom for quite a while. Sometimes not. Almost inevitably, I have time to open an e-mail, but as soon as I am absorbed, I hear the call. "Okay! I'm done!" What do I often reply? "Just a minute! I'm checking on something! *Just a minute!*"

I do hear myself. I'm talking about time. Time is such a shape-shifter for caregivers. On some days, I wonder, "Will this ever end?" On other days, especially those moments when I look at my much-loved husband, whose smile can still twist my heart, and notice how fragile he has become, I think of time differently. He is leaving me. We have so little time left together. Maybe only just a minute.

AT THE FOOT OF THE
ROLLER COASTER

September 20

I am sitting in the airport. I am shaking a little, not because my flight has been delayed or canceled but because I am here at all. Until the moment I walked through the arch at Security, I wasn't sure I'd get this far.

I have cashed in my frequent-flyer miles to finance a nine-day trip to London. My doctor and friends had been urging me to do it, to take a break that would enable me to continue James's and my other journey, the staggering march led by Parkinson's, to the end.

I am in the airport. Two weeks earlier, I returned from an afternoon of errands to find our aide Martha in an agitated flutter. James, she said, had abruptly collapsed. With help, he had walked down our long flight of outdoor steps to say good-bye to a visiting old friend, walked back up, and then, still with Martha's guidance, mounted a short flight of indoor stairs.

On the landing, his legs begin to wobble. She had been able to maneuver him the short distance toward his bedroom, so he had not actually crashed to the floor. He had seemed woozy and out of balance for half an hour afterward. Now he had recovered. When I hurried into the bedroom, he was sitting contentedly in his favorite chair, glancing at a box of old snapshots. He didn't appear alarmed by what had happened.

Martha and I conferred. I wondered about calling a doctor. Maybe 911? But Martha, an experienced practical nurse, said James had shown no signs of stroke, double vision, paralysis, or loss of consciousness. She decided he had suffered a muscle spasm in his hand, lost hold of the stair railing, panicked, and folded. I thought perhaps that Parkinson's, which slows or stops messages from the brain to the muscles, had simply "frozen" him for moments. (James has not yet had a classic episode of Parkinson's "freezing," which can cause a momentary inability to move.)

The next day, another aide, Amy, caring and competent, though not a nurse, came to spend the morning with James. Before heading out for a much-needed bike ride, I explained what had happened. I didn't expect this to recur, I told her, but just in case, she should remember that Parkinson's patients don't really crash to the floor. They crumple. If this occurred, she should hold onto James. She wouldn't be strong enough to hold him up, so she should simply sink gently to the floor with him. Then call me immediately, I said. As always, I'd have my cell phone at my waist. Amy told me she was sure they'd be fine.

I put on my helmet and took off. Feeling the wind whirl past my face was miraculous relief. I let something intangible but heavy slip off my shoulders, landing somewhere on the bike path behind me. Then my phone rang.

"James had another accident," Amy said a little tremulously. "But he's okay. He's not hurt, except when he went down on the front porch, he caught his bare arm on the edge of the metal mailbox. It's a long cut. I've bandaged it up." I asked a few quick questions. Had James been coherent? "Oh, yes," Amy reassured me. "The first thing he did was to ask if I was okay." That, I distractedly thought, was just like James.

I told Amy I'd pedal home as fast as possible. Expect me in

twenty minutes. Meanwhile, keep him comfortable. Don't try to get him up. You can't do it alone.

As I swung hard around the lake path—I'm sixty-nine and not the speediest cyclist, but I pumped my legs with crazy energy—I knew the weight had returned not only to my shoulders but into my heart and stomach. The goblin of Parkinson's always lives there, disappearing briefly—on a bike ride, for instance—but waiting in the shadows.

I also told myself, "Well, that takes care of London. Too bad, but tell yourself so what? You've been to London before. Chances are maybe you can go again someday. Keep your sense of proportion here. Not such a big deal. Not such a big deal. Not such a big deal." (However, I sometimes find it hard to keep a sense of proportion. James hates to hear me swear, but he wasn't there. As I was pumping my pedals, I did.)

What was a big deal: something serious was happening to James. Something new and awful in this unpredictable, progressive disease. Until now, James had been using stairs fairly well, as long as he could depend on a handrail and a reassuring pair of helping hands on his transfer belt, a heavy-duty adjustable wide band around his waist. Now I would have to call our family doctor, Eben. I would also need to contact our specialist, Dr. Sutton. I needed advice, fast.

Once home, I slammed off my bike, tore off my helmet, and dashed into our house. James, to my disbelief, was quietly lying on the living-room sofa. Twenty minutes ago, he had been flat on our front deck. Amy said quickly, "I did get him up. We got up together. We put our arms around each other's waists and just got up."

"Well done!" I almost shouted, and then I sat down by James. He looked tired, his bandage needed redoing (I'd never shown Amy how to tape his sensitive skin), but he sounded okay. He couldn't explain what had happened.

Hurrying to the kitchen telephone, I looked up Eben's beeper number and rang it. I'd only used it once before. He is a very busy doctor, and I don't take the privilege of that number lightly. Eben soon called back. I ran through symptoms and answered his questions. "No, this is not 911 time," he said calmly. "This sounds like another piece of Parkinson's. It is very likely that his blood pressure is tanking. I'll order a very low dose, just a smidgen, of something that might help stabilize that a little."

Then I e-mailed Dr. Sutton. From something Janet said months ago, I wondered if perhaps she might want me to change James's dosage of Sinemet, his basic Parkie pill. As with Eben's beeper, I am conscious of the privilege of having her e-mail address, which she had cautioned me last year she seldom gave out. I had used it twice. Now it was time again.

As I carefully composed my note to her, clear and specific, without dramatics, I found myself writing: "James has started to crumple unexpectedly." I stopped and stared at that word: crumple. That was what Parkinson's had become, a long process of crumpling. I pictured us both, James and me, shrinking, wavering, and slowly sinking to the ground, holding onto each other as best we could.

Dr. Sutton e-mailed me back almost immediately. She agreed with Eben's suggestion of a new medication and also proposed lessening James's Sinemet slightly. Then she went on: "In the larger picture, however, this is an ominous development. This does not usually happen until the very end of PD. Meanwhile I suggest you think about preventing his falls by keeping him in a chair or lying down."

For the next three or four days, James was so groggy in the morning that Martha and I had to swivel him from bed to his portable wheelchair, where we fed him breakfast from a tray table. He was unsteady on his feet. Only in late afternoon did he begin to recover his balance and some alertness.

I didn't think much about London. I had replied to Dr. Sutton's e-mail with one more question: should I cancel my trip to London in two weeks? I was sure the answer was clear.

But she e-mailed back: "I think you can probably go. James should be all right. But when you return, you will want to remain home for the duration. Three months? Six months? A year? We'll see."

Her words whirled around in my mind. "Duration . . . six months . . . a year . . . we'll see." I now felt completely untethered—and also, paradoxically, tethered very tightly. "Remain." No breaks. A year?

After five days, James woke up one morning with brightness in his eyes and a return of energy. Almost without assistance, he walked down the stairs to the breakfast table. Later in the morning, he asked eagerly, "Can I go for a walk now?" Martha and I decided to let him try his walker, just down our alley for a brief spell. We hung on to him from each side. He insisted on taking the walker almost around our entire block. He was very hungry at dinnertime, and he slept through the night.

James continued to do well. After several days of this recovery, I began to think about London again.

Every day I watched James closely. My nerves were on high alert. I told everyone who asked that I hoped I was going to London, that I wouldn't need to decide until the last minute, that I would make all preparations, but I might have to cancel them. I took time to read through all the clauses in the travel insurance brochure.

I have never liked roller coasters. When I was young, I went many times to the Iowa State Fair. I wanted to do what my friends did. So I rode the Tilt-a-Whirl, which made me dizzy; the Ferris wheel, which always seemed to stop when I was a thousand feet in the air; and a terrifying ride with individual cars that turned upside down. Only once did I try the roller coaster, and at the very top, I looked down and was sure I was going to die. I got off at the bottom, and I never got on a roller coaster again.

Now I was on another roller coaster. This time I couldn't get off. I tried to deal with my tension. I rode my bicycle. I took walks.

I breathed in and out, using my little biofeedback device. Still, at night I tossed and turned, thinking of James, thinking of myself, wondering what I should do. Go? Stay? Go?

My friends offered an opinion with one voice: "GO!" James's children and my aides were unanimous: "GO!" Our doctor Eben urged me: "GO!" He even offered to drive me to the plane.

Four days before I was due to leave, I had a routine extraction of earwax. I have never had any aftereffects from this procedure. The next day, as I was on my hands and knees, craning my neck and peering into a low bathroom cabinet to find a few travel containers, I began to feel dizzy. Was the little room too warm? I stood up. I felt dizzier. I went downstairs. I did not feel better. Whenever I moved my head, I felt as if I had just gotten off a roller coaster. A roller coaster. Of course.

"Martha," I said, without showing how scared I was, "I'm feeling just a bit dizzy. I think I'll lie down for a while." So I did. But whenever I got up, the vertigo returned. After an hour, I was really scared. I called Eben's beeper. "This time it's me," I said, when he returned my call. I told him what was happening.

After a brief interrogation, he said reassuringly, "I think you probably have benign postural vertigo disorder. It is not that uncommon, especially as we get older. It usually resolves itself. I'll tell you an easy maneuver you can try, and if necessary you could also see a physical therapist. But for now, take a motion-sickness pill and lie down."

Lying on my bed, watching the room whirl around me if I turned my head, I knew I would not be going to London. My vertigo lasted for four hours. I breathed in and out, counting breaths to calm myself. The room whirled. If I had been emotionally shaken before, now I was holding onto my roller-coaster bar with damp, sweaty palms. When my dizziness finally crept away, I moved around the house as if on eggshells. I did not dare even to look at my empty suitcase, let alone start to pack anything in it. Vertigo: wasn't that also a metaphor for my life?

At the end of the afternoon, I sat up long enough to call my ear doctor's office. Surely someone there knew all about this? Yes, the nurse said, of course. That was no problem. No problem at all. Although no one could see me the next day, I could come in the following day—forty-eight hours before my supposed departure for London. Oh, yes, she said, she was sure I could go.

Next day, I packed a little. When I finally saw the doctor, he ran me through some tests, turning my neck this way and that, peering into my ears, studying my eyes, checking my reflexes, even looking up my nose. He studied my balance while walking. To his surprise as well as mine, I think, he told me definitively I did *not* have BPVD. My vertigo? No discernible cause. Perhaps an unusual migraine?

Yes, he too said quite positively, I could certainly go to London.

Now I am in the airport. I still have one foot on the roller coaster. It has stopped for the moment. In nine days, it will start up again. I hope I will be ready to climb back on.

GRAVY

October 20

"Gravy," James said. "I like gravy." Then he paused.

Dr. Sutton waited a minute or two. Then she asked encouragingly, "Well, I like gravy too. But gravy on what?"

James looked at her pleasantly. "Gravy. I just like gravy."

I tried to keep a straight face. A few months ago, at one of James's regular checkups, she had noted his continuing weight loss. Two or three pounds were disappearing every few months. Before Parkinson's, James weighed 168 pounds (and at six feet and very fit, that seemed about right.) Now he was at 136. We clearly needed to talk about food.

"So, is he eating well?" Dr. Sutton asked me.

"Well," I said, circling around a prickly subject, "meals are really difficult. I know he needs to gain weight, so I try to fix high-calorie dishes, but if I ate what he eats, I'd balloon up very quickly. So basically I have to produce two different meals three times a day, and I don't have a lot of time to do that. I can't spend too long cooking. Also he has become increasingly picky. I never know from one meal to another what he'll eat, and he doesn't like some things he used to love. When I put a plate in front of him, I'm just hoping for the best.

"Besides that," I went on, picking up speed, "James has always had a phobia about weight—this goes back to a time before I knew him—so he seems to feel better if he leaves food on his plate. This can be very frustrating, because actually, I'm a very good cook."

Dr. Sutton smiled. She looked at James again. "So is she a good cook, James?" she asked.

James, for once, didn't hesitate. "Her mashed potatoes are lumpy," he said.

Dr. Sutton raised her eyebrows queryingly at me.

I was seething. Not too long ago, I loved cooking. I bought my first cast-iron stockpot when I was twenty-three, and over the years I kept adding to a collection of cookbooks. For a long time, though, I haven't opened one. I don't even have time to dust them.

"He is referring to a new recipe I tried a few days ago," I said evenly. "We went out for lunch last week at Spoonriver, his favorite restaurant, and he raved about a side dish of mashed potatoes whipped with cooked carrots and coconut milk. The owner, Brenda, whom James adores, gave me the recipe. But I don't have a commercial ricer, just an ordinary masher, and so yes, the potatoes were a little lumpy."

"Well, I suggest you stick to really simple foods," Dr. Sutton said. "Just fix his favorites." (Did she imagine I had been fussing with Peking duck or beef Wellington?)

That was when she asked James what he liked.

So she got her answer: gravy. James likes gravy.

Before Parkinson's, food was not a problem. James and I always enjoyed our meals together. I did most of the cooking, and he was an appreciative and congenial dinner partner. We talked, laughed, and often watched the *PBS NewsHour* at suppertime. Sometimes we played gin rummy over dessert. Afterward, James usually washed the dishes.

Now we still watch the *NewsHour*, but mostly to fill the emptiness of the supper hour. James cannot talk and eat at the same time, and in any case, he cannot actually talk much. He eats very, very slowly. Mealtime endures at least an hour.

I make a little conversation, but mostly I'm jumping up and down, adding ice to his water, cutting up his food, helping him scoop or stab with spoon or fork, often sliding the utensil into his mouth, warming up a plate or coffee that has grown cold, feeding him pills, and then clearing dishes, fixing his dessert, and hoping to get the kitchen clean before I have to take James upstairs for bed.

By 5:00 p.m. on any ordinary day, I am worn out. But that is exactly when I need to move into a higher gear. My aide has left. Supper looms. I need to keep James entertained (or perhaps resting) within eyesight, while I figure out what to put on the table. ("Just three hours," I tell myself. "I can keep going for three more hours. He'll be in bed in three hours.")

So at 5:00 p.m. I'm not waltzing around the kitchen with a light heart. I'm hoping. I'm hoping that whatever I've planned will appeal to James and that he will eat some, if not most, of it. I have a few tricks. Sometimes I lie. Last week, for example, I was rushing through Trader Joe's, heaping easy-to-fix foods into my cart, when I saw on the deli shelf a tempting, plastic-covered, ready-to-heat dish of eggplant Parmesan.

I knew James doesn't eat eggplant. He is usually suspicious of tomato sauce. He doesn't like cheese, except for a sprinkling of Parmesan. He also currently rejects mushrooms, coleslaw, onions, avocados, olives, sausage, berries (indeed all raw fruits except for ripe Colorado peaches and white grapefruit), most greens, anything with seeds, brown bread or any white bread that isn't toasted, cream soups, ravioli or any filled pasta—I'll stop here.

This pickiness, while not entirely new—he was never an omnivore—is not James's fault. Parkinson's can turn taste buds inside out. One day James will happily eat a dish of chicken fried rice, and the next day (pressed for time, I plan for leftovers), he will push the rice around on his plate and say, "This is not my favorite." He has other ways of expressing dislike: "This doesn't taste right." "I don't prefer this." "Where did you get this?" For someone who has a hard time articulating his thoughts, he is very clear about what he doesn't want to eat.

As I considered the eggplant Parmesan, I also knew that, for no particular reason, James distrusts Trader Joe's. (I love it.) It only opened in Minneapolis a few years ago, and James never shopped there. He wishes I would always buy our groceries from Lund's, an upscale local chain. He trusts Lund's. But I remembered that James always enjoyed Broder's, an excellent Italian deli restaurant quite close to our house. James has been known to eat Broder's lasagna. I plopped the eggplant Parmesan into my cart. I had a plan.

That night I heated up the eggplant Parmesan, divided it into two pieces, and slid it onto a plate. The sauce was so thick it covered the eggplant. I cut up James's portion into small bites. The eggplant was indistinguishable. It looked just like lasagna with ground beef. In fact, as I forked some into my mouth, I thought the concoction actually *tasted* rather like lasagna. I was home free. "Isn't this delicious lasagna?" I asked James innocently. "Not too much meat, but just enough." James nodded. "Pretty good," he said. "Where did you get it?"

"Oh, I picked it up at Broder's," I said smoothly. He nodded again, and he finished his whole serving.

Besides lying, I vent. I have been known—I'm ashamed to admit this—to snatch away rejected dishes and bang them down on the kitchen counter. I mutter cross remarks. Although our small galley kitchen adjoins the dining table, when I stand in front of the refrigerator, James can't see me. So I sometimes stand there, scowl, and stick out my tongue as far as it will go. I stand there, making nasty faces at the refrigerator until I feel better, and then I go back to the table.

"You need to see eating problems as a possible control issue," advises one of my caregiving manuals. (Why do I keep reading these books?) "Simply let your loved one eat whatever he wants. Don't urge food on him." This is undoubtedly excellent advice. But if you see your husband dwindling away, and you know that this loss of weight contributes to his overall decline, it is very, very hard to think to yourself, "Oh, what the hell. Let him lose another two pounds this week. It doesn't matter."

Another manual was quite stern: "Eat the same meal that your loved one eats. Make sure that you enjoy your time together at the table. Avoid tension. Aim for a happy supper hour." I would love to invite this writer over for a meal and ask her to cook, serve, and eat it. Both high-calorie and low-calorie versions, please. For several mornings, noons, and nights—say, a month or two—in a row. Then I'd ask her if she was planning to revise her book.

I do what I can. If I find a prepared dish James likes—for example, Lund's scalloped potatoes with cheddar cheese, not to mention with many additives, is almost always a hit—I ignore nutritional wisdom and serve it. I even keep more of it in the freezer. I stock gallons of vanilla and chocolate Häagen-Dazs ice cream, the only two flavors he'll now eat. I add cocoa, whipping cream, and sugar to his coffee, and I am so lavish with butter that his toast almost disintegrates in an aromatic pool.

I think I am slowly learning to be more patient. Mostly this is not because I've become a better person, but because James is so much further along in this progressive disease. Uncertain and bumpy as Parkinson's is, I am trying to accept that I can't do much to alter its inevitable course. If he eats less, he eats less. If I'm doing all I can, I have to let go. (I can still occasionally be found in front of the refrigerator, however, my face screwed up like a monkey's, tongue sticking out.)

Meanwhile, I've discovered Lund's own brand of poultry gravy. I buy it. The word "poultry" is deliberately vague, because the list of ingredients bears little resemblance to any gravy I've ever made. But hey, I can heat it up in the microwave, it smells good, and James loves it on mashed potatoes.

So far, I've avoided serving him just gravy.

HOME, ALONE

November 20

On this late autumn afternoon, a cold wind was whipping leaves from the trees. Under a low gray sky, a faint drizzle dripped steadily on the front steps. Our back door had just closed behind James and aide Martha, who was taking him to the dentist for a routine cleaning. I would have two hours alone in the house.

Two hours. In my house. All by myself. The last time this happened was another dental appointment—four months earlier. Because of James's increasing fatigue, fits of muscle weakness, and uncertain mental focus, he can no longer go out for lunch or any other prolonged excursion. In fact, I didn't know yet that James would return in two hours so depleted he would sleep half the next day, and I would realize that even James's trips to the dentist were now over. All I knew this autumn afternoon was that I had been given two quiet, rain-streaked hours. A treasured gift.

Last year, soon after my friend Dolores's husband died after a massive stroke, she told me, "The worst part is coming home to the empty house. I can't bear it. I put it off as long as I can. When I finally open the door, I break down. Everything, every room, our home, was ours. We created it all together. I just sink onto the sofa and start to cry. I cry for such a long time. You can't believe how awful it is." Some nights, Dolores told me, she packed an overnight bag and went to stay with her married daughter. "But then," she added, looking beyond me, "I have to go home."

So I know that my longing to have the house to myself— maybe for a whole day? two days?—holds the ominous promise implied in the adage "Be careful what you wish for. You may get it." That is the dark conundrum of caregiving: you want, and you don't want.

I have lived alone for only a few months of my entire life. After a dorm in college, then a graduate-school dorm, and finally one semester with a girlfriend in a shared apartment, I married my first husband. During that rocky marriage, we briefly separated several times. He left, I stayed. I remember how frightened I was at night, alone in an echoing house. Returning home in the day, I felt uneasy as I turned my key in the lock.

During one reconciliation, I got pregnant. After we divorced, I had our daughter, a lively toddler, in my house, so I was not really alone. When she was a teenager, I met and married James. I sometimes try to imagine our house without James in it. I can't. Like Dolores and her husband, James and I furnished, arranged, and lived in this house as a haven we both loved. We liked being together so much that neither of us wanted to be away from the other for any extended period.

Yet my days had spaces I kept for myself. Until Parkinson's bound him too tightly, James, even semiretired, was usually gone for many hours, settling into his old desk at his office or enjoying lunch with friends. I happily welcomed him home. Dolores has warned me: somewhere ahead, I have very hard lessons to learn.

At this time, even in our ample house, I cannot find a room where I feel free. I have no privacy. At any moment I may hear a tap on the door from a caregiver: "Where is James's new rash ointment?" "Do you think I can take James for a short walk?" "James wants to find his book about tugboats [or box of snapshots, or postcard from an old friend, or file of drawings]."

Infuriatingly, I cannot even shut the door of any room where

I am trying to hide. We own three cats. I have in fact spent all my life with one or two cats, but these days, perhaps because none of our current trio is a lap cat, I have often wished someone— a sweet, gentle old lady?—would swoop into our house and carry them all off to a loving home where they could live out their remaining years with the devoted attention they deserve. (Right now they don't get it from me.) Cats are territorial creatures. They hate being locked out. So if I shut my door, one or more will sit outside forever, scratching, meowing, scratching. "Let me in!" "What's going on in there?" "I know you're there!"

Of course I can sometimes leave my house. A few times I've taken my laptop to a neighborhood coffee shop. But people gather there, they talk and laugh, they bang in and out. I can look for an easy chair at my local library, but the expedition takes time. Also, even libraries aren't all that quiet these days.

Nothing is the same as sitting alone in my own house. This is my shell. I belong here. So does James. That is why I am fighting so hard to care for him at home. But now I need more than ever before to gather some of this space around me. I am crowded in a way I have never known before.

Before James's dementia, he would have understood. Years ago, when James and I were standing on a Pacific coastline, watching whales spouting on the horizon, he turned to me with a grin. "You know," he said, putting his arm around me, "if you were a whale, you would migrate in a pod of two."

After James and Martha had left for the dentist, I took a phone off the hook. An answering machine would pick up any messages. I turned off my cell phone. I felt a little guilty; what if Martha had to call me? But I did it anyway.

Upstairs, at my desk, was the usual pile of bills, notices to be filed, forms to be filled out, e-mails to be answered. I needed to start on today's laundry. We were low on skim milk (me) and heavy cream (James). Instead I lay down on the sofa, pillows behind my head, and listened to the rain. It was a very whispery, intermittent rain, but I could hear it. I also listened to the house. I am always listening for James: his call, his cry, his voice. I am on constant alert for the sound of his uncertain feet clanging against the metal rails of his new hospital bed. I am ready to be startled by his bell, a large brass one, clanging loudly enough to summon all the children in the neighborhood.

For the moment I was alone. I could hear the refrigerator humming and then plopping ice cubes into a plastic tray. The furnace gave out a low, reassuring growl. A cat wandered into the living room and settled at my feet. She began to purr. I twitched a little; I could sense muscles starting to let go. I found myself breathing more slowly and deeply. The rain pattered on the wooden deck. I reached out and picked up a book from the coffee table. I could plunge into a few chapters before James and Martha returned. I paused a few minutes, soaking in the sound of the rain. Then I began to read.

THROUGH THE HOSPICE DOOR

December 23

I always knew the door was there. Years ago, watching a friend slowly wither and die from ovarian cancer, I saw how peaceful she felt in her own bedroom, supported by hospice, as family, friends, and caregivers quietly came and went, talking to her, holding her hand, tending her. As Parkinson's gripped James ever more tightly, I hoped I too could care for him at home until the end, and I knew a hospice program might make that possible.

Although James and I are not yet at the absolute end—I also know as I write this that lightning could strike before I finish my sentence—I can make no binding promise, either to him or to myself, that I can keep him out of a hospital. But I can hope. That is why I have now entered James in the Fairview hospice program.

The night I returned three months ago from my mad dash to London, I realized in a flash that I urgently needed to make changes in James's living arrangements. The next morning I called Eben, our family doctor and dear friend, who said he would come to see us on Sunday, just a few days away. He and I sat alone in the upstairs bedroom while an aide stayed with James in the living room. Eben warned me—as would the hospice staff—that the course of Parkinson's was one of the most difficult diseases for anyone to predict. Still, having watched James's decline very closely, he also felt that hospice would now be a valuable resource for us. He said he would send in a referral the next day and also talk to the hospice's medical director.

Our first week of hospice care was something of a blur, filled with comings and goings, meeting the various members of our hospice team, discussing, note taking, completing forms. But almost immediately I could sense some of my burden shift a little. On our kitchen window, where I stick Post-its, I printed out my new instructions: "DO NOT CALL 911. ALWAYS CALL HOSPICE FIRST." I underlined the hospice phone number with bold red ink.

In my first conversation with Mary, our hospice nurse, I had asked nervously about how hospice would help care for James in case something happened. Such as, I said—my uppermost worry—a fall? A broken hip? Mary looked closely at me. "Well," she said carefully, "you would have two choices. You can call 911. An ambulance will come and take him to the hospital for major surgery. Then he would enter rehab, although, with his balance problems, he might never walk again." She paused. "Or," she said, "you call us. We would come immediately and make sure James was comfortable."

We were both silent for a moment. I thought of James's increasing dementia, his frailty, his need for reassurance, his eighty-four years. "I understand," I said. I knew what choice I would make. James would not go to the hospital. (Later, as I was talking to Eben, he said flatly, "James would probably never even make it through the operation.") Then I asked Mary about, for instance, pneumonia. "Right now," she said, "we would treat it with oral antibiotics." I heard the message in "right now." I understood that too.

Soon after we entered the hospice program, I had a startling example of what a help this would be. Because Fairview raises private money for its hospital foundation, its Medicare-based hospice can provide several extras, like occasional visits from a massage therapist or a music therapist and—this is huge—free delivery of medications.

Two weeks after signing up, on a late Friday afternoon, I had an unexpected bulletin from Martha, who called me to James's room. "I think James has a bladder infection," she said. (He had never before had one in his life.) All day, she said, he had been complaining about burning during urination. "Perhaps," Martha went on, "since Mary is coming today for her weekly visit, she might have a sterile container. We could get a clean catch. Then you could arrange for a test."

A "clean catch" would not be a simple or easy solution. Once, months ago, in Eben's office, James had been quite unable to provide such a specimen. I had no illusions he could now. Worse, I quickly thought ahead, even if we obtained a sample, this is Friday afternoon. Offices close. Bottle in our refrigerator. Monday I'd have to drive to Eben's lab. An hour round-trip. Leave sample, wait for results. So it would be Tuesday, maybe Wednesday. Meanwhile, what? I began to get a headache.

Soon Mary arrived. Martha explained James's symptoms and—she was quite blithe about this—the pending clean catch. (I thought for a moment of a trout jumping out of a stream; James used to love fly-fishing.) Mary gently interrupted her. "Oh, I don't think we want to wait for him to develop more symptoms," she said. "I have standing orders for quite a few prescriptions. I think"—she thought for a moment—"we'll start him on Cipro. Has he had that before?" He had. She picked up her cell phone, dialed, and said a few words to the pharmacist on the other end of the line.

"But I don't know how I can go out to the drugstore to pick that up," I said rather plaintively. "Martha is leaving soon, and then you'll be gone, and I can't leave James alone in the house."

"Oh, that's not a problem," Mary said reassuringly. "They'll deliver it."

Are you kidding? I thought. After hours? On Friday night?

Years ago, our local pharmacy delivered prescriptions, but only several days after filling them, and the store ultimately stopped that unprofitable service. Our health plan has a mail-order option, but that sometimes can take five to ten days. I sighed to myself and looked uneasily at James. Painful urination. Next, a fever? And then?

After Mary left, I fixed James supper. She had only been gone perhaps forty-five minutes when the doorbell rang. Rather cross, I got up from the table—another door-to-door solicitation, always at the dinner hour—and there stood a man with a small package and a tablet to be signed. "Your prescription," he said. "Sign here."

I was stunned. So I could start James on his antibiotic a few minutes later? Within two days, James felt better. A week later, cured. The moment I signed that prescription receipt, I was a true believer in hospice care.

Soon after Christmas, our hospice program will give us a ninety-day review. If James has improved, we might have to leave the program. James keeps losing weight and cognition, slowly, slowly, but inevitably. We won't flunk hospice. At the end of March, we'll have another review. I don't look that far ahead. All I can see is fog.

"Hospice" makes an ending seem imminent. It often is. Sometimes a patient is only in hospice for a few days before death; our Fairview program thinks that is usually not enough time for their services to be as useful as possible. For most hospice patients, I'm told, two months is an average length of stay. Of life. But Parkinson's is different. So when I mention to anyone that James is now in hospice care, I hastily add, "He is doing okay at the moment. This could last for a very long time."

Now I keep lecturing myself: Do not think of hospice as a waiting room. Do not play hide-and-seek with death. Do not try to penetrate that fog in the future. This is today; stay there.

TIME, AGAIN

December 24

Time, again. I have been writing this memoir, sporadically and unevenly, for almost a year. I do not go back and reread my entries, and who knows? Maybe I will never want to relive these past ten months. I know I have often written about time, its brevity, its compression, and its disappearance. Time blurs. Days of the week pass now without my always quite knowing which day it is—Wednesday? Thursday? I look at my big wall calendar, scribbled with notations and appointments, to steady myself. I want to keep my feet firmly planted on today.

Since James and I have entered our hospice program, time has morphed once again. Perhaps that sense of an approaching end, no matter how many months away, has made me listen differently to the voice that so frequently natters, complaining, in my head: "I wish I could drop in on Barb this afternoon, but I don't have time." "If only I could drive to the zoo one afternoon—I haven't been there for years—but I don't have time." "If I had time, I could join that gym with a swimming pool. Oh, I wish I could swim for just half an hour today instead of stomping around on these icy sidewalks." "I want to sit in my cushy yellow chair in the sunshine and read one of my piled-up new books, but I don't have time." "Will I ever play the piano again?" "Can I imagine ever cooking for friends again?" "Will I ever have time?" My entries here are filled with that voice.

Now I hear a response, as automatic as an echo. I am startled by how this echo—just one line, the last sentence of a novella by Katherine Anne Porter—has appeared in my mind. I read "Pale Horse, Pale Rider," the title story of a collection first published in 1939, at least forty years ago. Where has this line been hiding? I don't even remember the plots of some novels I read last month or the week before. Nor have I ever returned to this story.

(Just now, I hurried down to a basement shelf stuffed with dusty books. *Pale Horse, Pale Rider* was still there, its paperback spine cracking apart as soon as I opened the yellowing pages. I only wanted to make sure I was right about that line. I was.)

In this story two young people, Miranda and Adam, fall in love. The story takes place during World War I, at the height of the influenza epidemic that swept mercilessly through America. Adam is a soldier. Miranda and Adam meet when he is on leave, about to depart for the front. I remember their rapidly unfolding love story, tender and believable. They have discovered each other just in time. (There it is again: time.)

Miranda, however, becomes ill almost to death with the flu, and Adam faithfully nurses her. When she finally awakens, she learns that the war is over. She also learns that Adam has died of the influenza. As Miranda, dazed, considers her new future, she sees an utterly changed world around her. She thinks to herself— and this is the clear-eyed, devastating line that in its stark pain has stayed with me all these years—"Now there would be time for everything."

OFF THE BALANCE BEAM

January 15

I feel as if I am about to fall off my balance beam. I picture every caregiver on one, usually performing with an outward calm, like a confident acrobat, but concealing an inner terror: "What in the world will I do now?" For many of us this must require both courage and faith, because I am often dizzy and close to gasping as I edge my way forward. The balance beam hangs in an enveloping haze.

When James entered hospice, I imagined that the haze was lifting—revealing, I was sure, grief and desolation, but still a certain clarity about an ending. Parkinson's, however, has its own devastatingly inscrutable ways. Yes, James is worse. He no longer can mount the short flight of stairs for breakfast or for supper. At lunch he is usually fairly mobile, with help. His mind is much more hazy, his speech often incoherent. But his spirit seems indomitable, and his face still lights with pleasure when I come to help him out of bed in the morning. He is eating better, sometimes with gusto. No one knows what exactly will happen next, or when.

Only another long-term caregiver can truly understand the turbulent opposing forces, like buffeting winds, that rock my balance beam. As James smiles at me in the morning (awake too early!

too early!), I am filled with a tenderness that floods my heart. But later in the day—maybe only an hour later, as I'm trying to spoon his breakfast Cream of Wheat into his mouth, and he shuts his mouth too soon, and I'm dabbing with a damp paper towel at his oversized "apron"—I hear myself shouting inwardly, "Oh, Lord, how long? *How long?*"

That is the terrible ambivalence that shakes my balance. I sometimes dispassionately watch myself, like a visitor from the outside world, as I am straining every muscle to keep James from slipping to the floor before I complete his transfer from bed to wheelchair, or as I carefully floss his teeth, or as I put his fleecy hand warmers into the microwave to heat. (His hands are so icy now.) Together with my devoted team of aides, I know I am fighting as hard as I can to keep James alive, comfortable, and even happy. And yet . . . and yet.

"I have never known a caregiver, especially one who is dealing with dementia, not to feel ambivalence," Lonnie, our hospice social worker, told me not long ago. She spoke very softly and gently, as if she were comforting a child. "If you allow yourself to think 'I wish he would die!' you feel guilty not only at the time but also in advance, because you think you'll someday look back and feel even more guilty. But don't worry. All of your feelings are normal. What matters is what you are doing, not what you are thinking. You are doing a great job. Just be sure to try to be good to yourself as well." I wish I knew exactly how.

WHATCHA KNOW, JOE?

January 16

I used to know stuff. Lots of stuff.

When I graduated from high school in 1957, I had memorized almost all the lyrics to every song Frank Sinatra ever recorded. Sinatra has stayed with me. As my long-distance daughter and I were recently doubling up on a Sunday *Times* crossword over the phone, I spotted a Sinatra clue. I was incredulous that she had never heard one of his classics. I then warbled the whole bleak song to her in my slightly off-key, one-octave voice: "Make it one for my baby and one more for the road . . . that long, long road." As I sang, I heard the lyrics in a new way. A love song and a long, long road.

Oh, I once knew stuff. When I was a worried graduate student at Berkeley, facing a legendary ninety-minute oral exam, I was warned about what the three examiners might ask. One professor liked to demand: "Date Pope's canon." This required a quavering student to recite all the titles and publication dates of major works by poet Alexander Pope (1688–1744). I was temporarily able to do this, although that particular memory feat lasted maybe a week or less.

I knew other stuff, too. My first husband was an avid fan of the Minnesota Twins. So I too became a fan. For a few years in the 1960s, when the Twins were a sparky, feisty team heading toward a World Series, I followed their games, occasionally in the ballpark, otherwise on radio or television. I studied their stats. I could tell you batting averages, runs batted in, pitching records, strikeouts. (Oh, Harmon Killebrew! Tony Oliva! Rod Carew! César Tovar! I miss you!)

These days I feel I don't know anything. Friends, even acquaintances, ask me thoughtful and caring questions, and I have no answers to give them.

Question: "If James is in hospice, does that mean the end is near?"

Answer: "I don't know."

Question: "But don't your doctors have some idea?"

Answer: "It's just a guess. Hospice is intended for a six-month limit, but it can be extended."

Question: "As James continues to get worse, do you really think you can keep him at home?"

Answer: "I hope so, but I don't know."

Question: "Do you plan to stay in your house afterward?"

Answer: "For a while. I don't know."

Question: "If you do move, have you thought about where you'd like to go?"

Answer: "I've thought about it, but I don't know."

Question: "Would you want to travel again?"

Answer: "Probably, but I don't know."

Question: "Will you write again?"

Answer: "I don't know."

I don't know, I don't know, I don't know.

As I lay in bed this morning, thinking about all these questions with no answers, I remembered something. Since James served in World War II, we used to quote snatches of songs and jingles from that era. At that moment, I could almost hear James murmuring: "Whaddya know, Joe? I don't know nuttin'!"

All day I kept hearing that refrain in my head. "Whaddya

know, Joe? I don't know nuttin'." It wouldn't stop. I started wondering where it came from and what were the rest of the words. Who said it? Where? When? (A caregiver can obsessively focus in order to force other thoughts out of one's mind.) After supper, I thought I'd better put this question to rest. I consulted Google.

For the first time ever, Google failed me. No matter which combination of words I tried, nothing worked. Without ever learning the source of this ditty, I only found repetitions of the anonymous phrase in different contexts. After a while, Google gave up and notified me that I had just seen all the significant results.

I gave up too. It's not just me. Even Google doesn't have the answers to every question. I could start answering some of my inquirers with a give-it-up shrug and two sentences: "Whaddya know, Joe? I don't know nuttin'."

[Much, much later, after writing this chapter, I learned that Google was in fact all-knowing. A more clever searcher discovered that the actual song runs, "Whatcha know, Joe? I don't know nothin'." I indeed knew nothing.]

OBSESSIONS

January 22

I need to find a new obsession.

I first discovered how useful an obsession could be many years ago. James (who could still go to movies then) and I held hands, as we always did at movies, while we watched *Walk the Line,* a romanticized but emotionally powerful biography of the young Johnny Cash. I was fascinated.

How had I almost forgotten that deep, hypnotic voice, with its accompanying heavy beat, BOOM CHICKA BOOM, BOOM CHICKA BOOM? When I was a teenager, I'd avidly listened to his great hits, not just the movie's title song but others like "Folsom Prison Blues," "Ring of Fire," and "Rock Island Road." For most of my years growing up, the Rock Island ran through Ames to Chicago, and returning from college in the East, I rode three trains to get home. When I finally transferred to the Rock Island in Chicago, I could hear that song beating in my heart as the wheels clicked and clanked: "The Rock Island Line is a mighty good road . . . Get your ticket at the station for the Rock Island Line."

I came back from that movie wondering why I didn't know more about Johnny Cash. So I sent for the latest biography. I quickly learned that the movie—which ends so happily, with Cash freed from his years of addiction and rejoicing in his family life—was not, of course, the entire truth. Cash lapsed back into addiction, he had extramarital affairs, his son and stepchildren were not trouble-free, he broke angrily with his yearslong friend and guitarist Marshall Grant, and his popularity developed (and surmounted) jagged valleys.

Now I was really hooked. Who was this complicated man? Was it possible to know? I ordered Marshall Grant's book about Cash, then a biography of June Carter Cash by their son (she too had struggled with drugs), even a ghosted memoir by his first wife, Vivian, who felt her truth also needed to be told.

At the same time I bought Cash songs and albums. Not every song was riveting, but I listened to them all, hymns, folk, rock-and-roll ballads, blues, railroad sagas, everything. In our car, when I drove us down to our Wisconsin retreat, I played them over and over. James was tolerant. In fact, he laughed when I regaled him with my own (unaccompanied) version of "Long Black Veil," its melodrama belted out at the top of my lungs. Something about the darkness of Cash's story—shot through with light too, and illumined with his unwavering belief in redemption—was just what I needed to absorb then. I was beginning to glimpse the encroaching darkness myself.

During this obsession—and I still play Cash songs sometimes—I could easily slip away for an hour or more from what I knew was going on in my life. At night, after James was in bed, I could pick up a book and reenter Cash's life. At those times, I could lock onto Johnny Cash, not James.

Since I have spent much of my life disappearing into books, finding obsessions there was not difficult. After years of scoffing at mystery/thriller fans, I discovered I had begun to flip eagerly on Sundays to Marilyn Stasio's *New York Times* column, Crime. I had no patience with many best-selling authors, whose writing seemed pedestrian, but Stasio introduced me to a clever few whose serial novels—I like a writer whose work I can follow obsessively from one book to the next—were literate and intriguing.

That was how I took up with Carol O'Connell, who writes with wit and panache about a female detective, Mallory, who is young, gorgeous, brilliant, and rageful. Mallory's mysterious history reveals itself slowly throughout the novels. I started somewhere in the middle of the series, retraced my steps, and then continued voraciously.

About the time I discovered O'Connell, Stasio also led me to Lee Child. I felt that my rapid addiction to Lee Child was a guilty secret, because his sleek, polished thrillers about Jack Reacher, an impossibly strong, ingeniously resourceful, and utterly cool ex-military man, often erupt into the gory violence I always avoid in movies or most books. But I admired Child's prose, in which every sentence is pared down to a snappy minimum. Most of all, I was captivated by his hero, who could single-handedly and dexterously take on vicious enemies who always outnumbered him. I knew Reacher would survive. He was all-powerful. I didn't need a psychologist to tell me why, at this time in my life, such a hero was appealing.

When I finally admitted this obsession to a friend (and only one!), she startled me by saying that she too fanatically read the Reacher novels. "Do you know what you've become?" she asked. "Look at the fan Web site. You'll find you are now a Reacher Creature!"

A Reacher Creature. This is where obsessions can lead.

Diving into these unexpected, but very useful, indulgences, I would sometimes feel regretful, when I emerged, that perhaps I had wasted my time. After all, I have always been very picky about literary quality in books. I understandably think a great deal about time these days. So I decided to begin to read certain classics that I'm sure my graduate school teachers, not to mention my own students, always assumed I had.

Homer's *Odyssey*, for example. I probably first encountered it in the golden age of Classics Illustrated, comic books I devoured when young with the same hunger as I did *Modern Screen* and

Photoplay. Then, as I gradually roamed through English literature, I garnered enough episodes from the *Odyssey* to glimpse the whole story. I just had never read the epic poem from start to finish.

This, I thought, would be a worthwhile obsession. True, I didn't reach for the *Odyssey* at night as ardently as I did O'Connell or Child. But I did find that I was enjoying myself. Yes, it soon occurred to me, this *is* great! Why did I wait so long? When I was done, I felt I had been edified and nourished, not simply entertained. So I virtuously ordered a few other classics. My must-read-soon bookshelf now holds *The Iliad, War and Peace, Don Quixote,* and Dante's *Inferno*.

When I do finally get James to bed, though, not much of my brain is functioning at top speed. I bogged down halfway through Dante, and I keep meaning to pick it up again. But I haven't. Yet. I look at my bookmark sticking out of the volume and reassure myself: Just Not Yet.

For a short time, I thought I could obsess about reading all ten of the *New York Times Book Review*'s Best Books of the Year. The list came out last month. I finished one. But I have found that it is not healthy for me right now to tackle books whose reviews or dust jackets include the following words: war, abuse, incest, drugs, alcohol, degradation, depression, despair, torment, mortal, shocking, brutal, bleak, unflinching. These days, I flinch too easily.

Our postman, Paul, who is bright and funny, asked me curiously not long ago, as he handed me yet another book-size package, "Do you actually read all these books?" Caught, I smiled a little. "No," I told him, "but I want to. They give me something to look forward to." He nodded. He knows what is going on in our house.

I can't pretend that all, or even most, of my obsessions are high-minded. Since its beginning I have been nuttily devoted to the medical soap opera *Grey's Anatomy*. A one-hour drama with multiple continuing threads of plot, it can whisk me away from reality quite nicely. I like to have two or three such shows—a few escapist hours—to anticipate each week, so I am always searching for an additional one. So far I have lost *Shark* and found *The Good Wife* and *The Mentalist*. Whatever will I do when *Grey's Anatomy* ends?

Another great source of distraction is eBay. When one of my caregivers reported with dismay that she had accidentally dropped one of my old Limoges soup bowls, the antique ones with little pink flowers that I love, I quickly reassured her. I had, after all, bought it very inexpensively on eBay. "Don't worry," I said, already looking forward to a few stolen minutes at my computer, "I'll just find another one like it." Unfortunately, I again have plenty of soup bowls. I can't think of anything on eBay that I need right now. What I do need, eBay doesn't sell.

I frequently find Google an easy escape. Who was that actor I remember in *To the Lighthouse*? How tall was Paul Newman? Is Billy Graham (with Parkinson's) still alive? What happened to Piper Laurie? Does Bob Dylan have children? Once answered, however, these dazzlingly unimportant questions no longer hold possibilities.

Looking around my house, I can certainly find short-term opportunities for concentration. When I can't stand looking at streaks of dust and moldy containers on a kitchen shelf anymore, I have been known to take a precious hour to clean it out. I really focus for that hour. But this housekeeping mood doesn't strike often. In fact, it will likely lie dormant for months. In my closet, only weeks ago, I folded, color-coded, and stacked my T-shirts. I sorted my socks and threw out the ones that didn't match. I hung up belts. Very satisfying. But I am now tired of my closet.

Last fall, when I knew hospice was approaching, I obsessed for weeks about making James's lower-level room, once my daughter's, cozy and welcoming. Using hours plucked from here and there, I worked on this for many days. I rearranged furniture, installed caregiving supplies, set up a TV, fixed a DVD player, changed pictures, piled up colorful pillows, and even sewed a bright corduroy cover to slip over the ugly metal front panel of his hospital bed.

At my request, a friend who is a professional painter slapped a coat of muted purple on the rust-streaked legs of the card table where James now eats. I laid a bright, block-print cloth on top. I found a jewel-toned paisley shawl to drape over James's commode in the daytime. The room looks as cheerful as possible. But it is done.

Obsessions come and go. They serve an essential purpose, and then they vanish.

So where is my new obsession? I am already anxious to find one. I am sure it will appear. As with so much in my life right now, I can only wait.

THE LAST CHRISTMAS

January 31

Of course I don't really know if this was the last Christmas. Despite James's entry into hospice in early October, he is still walking (a little), eating (some), and showing awareness (spotty and subdued) of his increasingly small world. I think sometimes of Dylan Thomas's much-anthologized poem to his dying father: "Do Not Go Gentle into That Good Night." Thomas urges, "Rage, rage against the dying of the light." James is not raging. I am not even sure that he knows the light is slowly fading; he has never spoken of dying. I can't tell how much he is able to hold in his Parkinson's-riddled brain. James will go gently, I think, because he has retained his inner sweetness. But he loved life intensely, and he will not slip away easily.

Now, in late January, this past Christmas seems as if it happened a year ago. As I was slogging through the holidays, which seemed both ragged and interminable—caregivers needing time off, snow and ice clogging our driveway and walks, Christmas cards piling up to be answered in months (if at all), a few essential presents wrapped—I thought from time to time, "I will probably be alone next Christmas."

Thinking "This is our last Christmas" left me numb rather than sad. Our past few Christmases have not been very festive. I have to let my mind slip back at least six years to a holiday (shared with dear friends, far away, in New Zealand) where I felt relaxed and celebratory. This year I decided to concede only one modest decoration to the holiday, a small pot filled with evergreen branches that gave a convincing impression of a real Christmas tree. One of James's daughters decorated it for me. It was quite charming, actually, wreathed in fairy lights that turned on at the first sign of dusk and glittery with a set of suitably tiny ornaments. Still, I could barely muster enough enthusiasm on Christmas morning to open the presents a few friends and family had insisted on. ("No presents this year," I'd protested in vain.)

Looking back, beyond Christmas, I see that the realization "This is our last . . ." or "This is James's last . . ." rarely occurs to me at the time. Only later do I understand that he will not go to another movie, he will not go out to lunch again, he is unlikely to drive with me to any of our favorite places—or, in fact, anywhere.

When I recall the sweep of our twenty-eight years together, I feel both a rush of gratitude and a blast of grief. Two recurring images tend to flash into my mind. In the first, James and I are on one of our many trips to Britain, and we are setting out midmorning for another day's adventure. James slides comfortably into the right-hand driver's seat—he was always a confident driver—as I settle myself next to him, maps on my lap, brochures in a satchel at my feet. "So where are we going today?" he asks eagerly. "I hope we're going to see another garden."

"Oh, we certainly are," I say, as I pull out *The Good Gardens Guide* from my satchel. I tell him what wonders to expect when we get there. "Then," I add with anticipatory gluttony, "we can stop for a great lunch at a country-house hotel that's listed in *The Good Food Guide*. If we have time, I thought afterward we could take in a ruined abbey not far away."

"Of course we'll have time," James says.

For a while we did have time. Then we didn't. Five years ago, as our plane left London, after I looked back on a rewarding but very difficult ten days there—James's gait was already tentative, and he almost crashed once as he navigated the steps of a London bus—I remember thinking, "This is our last trip to England." Never again would the two of us walk hand in hand along the Thames or ramble into the countryside.

My other image is more recent. Last May, I drove James to our Wisconsin retreat, which he designed for us twenty-five years ago and which had been our refuge and delight for all those years. In "Beige Lies, Pink Lies, Purple Lies," I described how, to my dismay, James was seized by terrible anxiety and disorientation for two nights and how I had to take James home as quickly as possible.

What haunts me now, more than eight months later, are those last moments before we left. As we walked carefully to the car after breakfast, my hand gripping his arm, his other hand trembling on his cane, James stopped. In front of the car, he was pausing to look out once more at my rambling, messy, and extravagant garden and two striking, very small outbuildings, which were among his last architectural creations. Leaning on my arm and his cane, he said thoughtfully, "I like that roof peak. I think this summer I will take pictures of some details around here and make an album of them." (For a modernist architect, Mies van der Rohe's dictum "God is in the details" is almost a scriptural quotation.)

I already knew James would never return to this place he loved so much. That beautiful spring morning we were standing only a few yards from a small half-covered deck, a minipavilion, which James called the "Garden Overlook," just big enough to hold two Adirondack chairs. James loved to sit there and watch me fervently pulling weeds and carefully patting down mulch. I wanted very much to lead him gently through the narrow arch of the Overlook and lower him into one of the chairs. I could sit in the other. We could breathe in the beauty of the garden. One last time.

But I had been up all night. I was disintegrating. I had a two hours' drive ahead of me, and I was running on nerve alone. So I helped James into the passenger seat, fastened his belt, stowed his cane, and got behind the wheel. I steered almost blindly down our gravel drive. I thought if I looked back my heart would break.

I still wish I had let James sit a while on the Overlook.

If he were reading this entry, which he never will, James would not want me to end on a note of heartbreak. I think he would prefer that I tell another story about last times, in which he is, I think, quite a hero. My own recklessness that day now makes me shudder.

On a recent wintry Saturday afternoon, when I escaped to a movie matinee, I left James in the care of Trish, a skilled and gentle young nurse who returns his open affection. He could enjoy an afternoon with Trish, and I with Colin Firth. But when I left the movie and turned on my cell phone, I could see a missed call from home. Trouble.

I called immediately. Trish was indeed in a pickle. Our house, tall and narrow, has several levels. James now lived and slept in what was once my daughter's room, ground level, two flights down from the master bedroom. James designed our upstairs bedroom with three wide, carpeted steps leading to a separate cozy space with three treetop windows. This nook holds two oversized, comfy, bright-yellow chairs. James always preferred the one under the largest window.

This small space has been one of James's favorite places to read, rest, or listen to music. We refer to it as the "Yellow Chair," as in, "Would you like me to take you up to the Yellow Chair?" Although James was now subject to leg crumpling—usually brought on by a devastating lack of confidence when he stumbled a little—on good days, when he was walking strongly, he could still be helped those two flights of stairs to the Yellow Chair. I had long ago installed handholds (large brass drawer handles) on a low wall beside the three carpeted steps in the bedroom. Once he sank into his chair, someone piled supporting pillows under and around him because he had difficulty getting up from such soft, low cushions. James could nestle there, happily surveying his domestic domain.

"James was walking quite well," Trish reported on the phone, her voice a little shaky, "and he really wanted me to take him up to the Yellow Chair. So I did. But almost as soon as he sat down, he fell asleep. When he woke up, he was so groggy he couldn't stand very well. Then he lost his footing and panicked. He is too wobbly now even to get his balance. And of course we can't try those three stairs either. How soon will you be home?"

"Twenty minutes," I said. I drove home as fast as the snow-packed street allowed. "Okay, the cavalry is here!" I yelled when I rushed in the back door.

(I was overconfident.)

I ran up the stairs to the bedroom. Trish had managed to maneuver James to his commode-chair, which she had hurriedly carried up from downstairs, but now they were stuck. "I didn't dare leave him again to go all the way down to his room and grab the portable wheelchair, because he might try to get up and fall," Trish said apologetically.

"I can get that," I told her, and in minutes I had brought his lightweight, sturdy wheelchair upstairs. But now the cavalry faltered. Although Trish and I were able (though not easily) to move James from the commode into his wheelchair, I could see that we two could never maneuver that wheelchair, with James seated in it, down those first three carpeted steps, not to mention the two other flights of stairs. We tried several times to get James to hold onto both of us, one on each side, so he could stand and walk, or possibly grab the handhold on the wall as we supported him. Even at his diminished 130 pounds, he was too much for us. He collapsed back into his wheelchair.

My mind raced over possibilities. My last resort would be the Fire Department. A nurse told me long ago I could make a nonemergency call to 911: "Be sure to say this isn't an emergency! Then ask for a lift assist. Two strong guys will come out, free of charge, and they'll hoist him up from the floor."

The nurse wasn't sure whether they would arrive in a shiny red fire truck. I cringed at the picture of that fire truck parked in front of our house, passersby gathering at the foot of our front steps, cars stopping, neighbors' doors opening. Of course I should have called the Fire Department. But I didn't.

First, I decided, "Frank!" James's son, who lives not too far away, is always willing to help, but at the moment, I discovered, Frank wasn't answering his cell phone. Probably he was on a long winter walk, which he likes to do on weekends.

Weekend! That meant that perhaps Rog, next door, young and vigorous, might be home, unless he and his wife had taken their two young children on an outing.

We were in luck. Rog was home, and he said he'd be over in moments. I met him at the door, explained the situation, and he walked into our bedroom with courteous aplomb. "Hello, James," he said politely. James smiled back. I introduced Trish.

The three of us tried to crowd around James and together lift him from his chair and support him, but we couldn't. "Well," I said a little dubiously, "I think we could maybe belt James into the wheelchair, Trish and I could take the front wheels, and Rog could grab the back handles. At least maybe we can maneuver him down these three steps to the part of the bedroom that has a bed."

"Let's try it," said Rog cheerfully. We took our positions, and slowly, bumpily, nervously, we edged James's wheelchair down the wide stairs. James called out once, "Watch it!" but he didn't flail around or grab at any of us. He was game.

Once on the main bedroom floor, we consulted. Could we now manhandle this wheelchair down not just one but two flights of steep, narrow stairs to James's room? I'd always thought of those flights as relatively short, but now they seemed impossibly long.

I knew what might happen. If one of us lost a grip or James

shifted and struggled so that we in turn lost our balance, we might all go tumbling down to broken bones or worse. But so far, so good. (I still cannot believe I did not call the Fire Department.)

"Okay," I said, "next flight." As we struggled awkwardly in the narrow width of the staircase, advising each other ("Hold it a minute!" "Slow now!" "Just two more steps!"), James tilting a little as we bumped down step by step, I thought of what a screwball picture we must make: James, rather dazed but sitting uncomplainingly in an unsteady, bouncing, precariously poised wheelchair as I grabbed one wheel; Trish, who was voicing concern about the strain on my shoulder, grabbing the other; and Rog, intensely concentrating on his lead position, thumping down the stairs. We were jammed together into a space configured for only two (thin) people passing each other. Bounce, thud, grunts. More shouts: "Wait!" "Almost!" "Hold on!"

One stair at a time. Very slowly. We did it. Once down to James's room on the ground level, we cheered and high-fived each other. James looked wrung out. I felt that way too. I gave Rog passionate thanks and a big hug, and then he hustled back to his waiting family. Trish and I looked at each other.

Taking her aside for a moment, I said, "You know, I hate to say this, but I really think that was James's last trip up to the Yellow Chair."

Trish nodded vigorously. "No question," she said.

I stood there, catching my breath. I wasn't going to obsess about this last time. I was simply going to accept the welcome fact that James was safe.

Not all facts are welcome, but there they are.

SILVER ANNIVERSARY

February 10

Yesterday was our silver anniversary. James and I have now been married for twenty-five years. We "kept company," as my mother might have said, for three years before that. Twenty-eight years together. And still counting.

Because we married (each for the second time) when I was forty-four and James was fifty-nine, I knew I could never look forward to a golden wedding anniversary. But by then, after eleven single years following my divorce, I had almost given up hope for a happy marriage. Twenty-five years together has been a miracle.

Our anniversary was a silvery day, with a gray but luminous sky reflecting the cuttingly sharp white of a new snowfall. Mounds of snow are heaped outside our door and windows; they line our sidewalks. When James looks out from his bed, all he can see is gray and white. I do not think he cares. He sometimes asks to have someone close the blinds because the reflected light is too bright.

He was in bed almost all day. During the past two weeks, James's Parkinson's seems to have seeped so deeply into his mind, drawing him down into its unfathomable depths, that he cannot easily awake in the morning. Some days he sleeps as if drugged, mouth open, snoring sonorously, until close to noon. He eats a late breakfast or lunch in bed. Martha or one of our other valiant aides can usually coax him up and into his shower in the afternoon—though not always. By 5:00 p.m., when I serve him supper, he is longing to return to bed, and by 6:30 p.m. he is gratefully flat on his back again, unable to turn from side to side, his eyes closed, his mind shut down.

When I went into his room in the morning, nudging him awake just long enough to give him a Sinemet pill, I told him that this was a very special day. Our twenty-fifth anniversary. He smiled and fell back into sleep.

At noon, as I was staring out my own study window, looking at the snow (and wondering if it would ever, ever melt), my phone rang. A dear friend, whom I haven't seen in six years, was calling from New Zealand, where we first met. Despite a ten-year difference in our ages, we share a very rewarding friendship, even if we don't speak or write for weeks or months. Shirley had no idea she had chosen to call on our silver anniversary. Talking to her, telling her what was happening and how I was feeling—she was once a caregiver—was like an unexpected celebration.

Later in the afternoon, when I made one of my periodic checks on James, Martha told me that he had been restless and nervous most of the afternoon. He would sink into sleep, talk and cry out, sometimes with fear, and then return to sleep. "Just a while ago," she said, "he suddenly woke up and said he thought he had died."

I was shocked. Although I have given him many openings—gentle, quietly permissive—to talk about what lies ahead, he has never spoken the words "death" or "dying." Even when Parkie had only slightly dulled his mind, he did not want to discuss endings. Some years ago, after Parkie had made a side entrance onto our stage, but was not yet commanding it, I printed out two copies of living wills and sat down with James to talk about their provisions. Mostly I suggested, and he agreed. He was clearly not comfortable dwelling on any of it.

So yesterday, when I heard his comment about dying, I asked Martha to give me some time alone with James. She left the room, and I sat on the edge of his bed and held his hand. Although he kept looking around the room as if he were searching for something, he seemed more alert than he had been all day. So I talked to him a little about our anniversary, how lucky we'd been, and how we would drink a few sips of wine in a toast at suppertime. (We did.)

Then I asked James about this hallucinatory dream. "Do you think you're dying?" I asked. I summoned courage to say the word. He looked at me and half-smiled. Then he said, "Possibly." He looked, unfocused, around the room. I waited. I probed very little, not much at all, because he didn't want that—I could tell—and then I said, "Well, don't die today. It's our twenty-fifth anniversary, and I couldn't stand remembering that."

"Okay," he said, and fell back asleep.

I called our hospice nurse, Mary, who will come today for a visit, but she reminded me that as long as he is eating and drinking (which he is), the end is probably not imminent. "But things can change on a dime," she said. I know that too.

After his supper, when Martha had left, I went into James's room. He had almost instantly fallen asleep. As I always do at his bedtime, I leaned over and whispered in his ear, "Good night. I love you." He can't talk much at all now, but he mumbled something, probably his usual "Me too." Then he paused and added very clearly, "With all my heart." In moments he was asleep again.

I sat in the dark next to the hospital bed and listened to his breathing.

THE NET IS LARGER THAN
YOU IMAGINE

February 28

> *It is always darkest before the dawn.*
> *God never gives us anything that we can't handle.*
> *Whatever doesn't kill you makes you stronger.*
> *This can be a time of tremendous personal growth.*
> *Live your life fully in the present.*
> *Treasure each moment.*
> *Count your blessings.*

Caregivers hear them all.

We accumulate every single cliché and bromide, although I surmise very few of our well-wishers have ever been long-term caregivers. As I just wrote "bromide," I couldn't help thinking of Bromo-Seltzer, as if, like an antacid, all these little sayings were supposed to bubble up inside me and soothe a constant ache. So far I have resisted answering, "Of course, and I also know the ones about how every silver lining has a cloud, and everything looks darkest just before it goes totally black."

Yet I admit I am humbled these days when my skeptical assumptions are unexpectedly overturned.

Many weeks ago, a friend sent me a supportive note, ending,

"The net is larger than you imagine." I began pondering: where was my net? Because I had been so satisfied with my long, happy, and companionable marriage, I didn't weave a wide net beyond it. I do not belong to a particular church. I am not a member of a book club, a garden club, a bridge club, or indeed any club at all. I don't like parties, and I haven't really entertained for years. I have a few close friends, but several now live in distant states or countries.

Last fall, Rachel, a visiting friend (one of those who moved away), and I reconnected for lunch. We were talking about how hard it seemed at our age to make new close friends. "I ask myself sometimes," I told her, "now that James is unable to do it, who in the world would take me to a colonoscopy and then wait to take me home?" We laughed. Rachel said, "Well, of course I would, if I were here. But that's a good point. *Who* in Santa Barbara besides my husband would take me?" We agreed that we both needed to work harder to find friends who could pass the Colonoscopy Test.

So at first I couldn't quite believe my friend: "The net is larger than you imagine." Then, not long afterward, I was reading in Mary Karr's memoir, *Lit,* about her embrace of Catholicism. Early in her conversion, she asks another well-known writer if he believes in God. He tells her, rather evasively, that he does sometimes give thanks. She decides that he must believe, because he thinks Someone or Something is listening to him.

This idea lingered in my mind. I pictured myself on a typical night, utterly drained, almost literally falling into bed. I want to fall asleep as soon as possible so that even if I wake, disturbed by racing thoughts or fears at 3:00 or 4:00 a.m., I can still get enough rest to make it through the next day. Giving thanks? For what?

But I didn't forget the idea. Several nights later, a few minutes before pulling the blanket around my ears, I decided to consider this. What could I think of? Almost immediately I remembered how grateful I'd been earlier that day when Tony, my trusted auto mechanic, had taken my ten-year-old car right into his shop, ignoring his crowded waiting lot. Tony knew I was hoping to drive the next day to our wooded retreat, a two-hour drive each way, and I was worried about my battery, which seemed sluggish. Not too long ago, Tony had revived that battery. Now he decided it was nearly dead and quickly replaced it. "I'd never let you drive all that way with a bad battery," he said, putting his arm around me. "Hey, kid, you always know I'm here if you need me."

Then I remembered that soon afterward I'd walked into the nearby consignment store where Tony's wife, Kim, works part-time. Because I wanted to stop risking my life on ice-packed sidewalks, I had finally joined a health club. So I needed a new swimsuit. I hate trying on swimsuits almost as much as I hate flossing James's teeth. Every suit I tugged on—the store didn't have many— seemed shockingly skimpy, slashed upward and downward to my navel, and was horrifyingly unflattering. I needed one *now*. I emerged from the dressing room looking quite defeated.

"Any of them work?" Kim asked. I shook my head. Kim, who is tall and gorgeous, understood. All women know about swimsuits. She motioned me over to the counter, leaned across it, and whispered, "Check out Marshall's. I happen to know they just got in their spring shipment of swimsuits." Half an hour later—the mall is only ten minutes away—I headed home with an attractive, comfortable swimsuit that didn't make me look like a pork roast.

Thanks for Tony. Thanks for Kim. And thanks for my home-made fish soup tonight. With pesto from last summer. All from my freezer. Thanks for my freezer. A few hours ago I had actually enjoyed supper.

This is a new development: a meal without stress. Not long ago, I had a revelation. (Revelations for caregivers are sometimes just solutions we've avoided seeing.) I could no longer navigate through the supper hour. My late-afternoon routine had finally bent me to a snapping point. Soon after 4:30 p.m., I had to hastily prepare a meal upstairs (while watching James downstairs on my monitor), dash up and down every few minutes to reassure him I was coming soon, carry both our meals downstairs, serve him by 5:00 p.m. because he took more than an hour to eat and was desperate for bed before 7:00 p.m., and then feed myself in quick gulps while slowly and patiently spooning food into James's mouth, cleaning when necessary. Then I had to carry up the dishes (to wash later) and go back downstairs immediately to prepare James for bed. Even as I write this, I feel breathless.

I remember saying to James that January night, in a near-hysterical voice, "I don't think I can do this anymore." He looked puzzled. I hurriedly changed the subject, but I started thinking. Why couldn't I ask Martha, our main aide, if she'd like to be paid to stay an extra hour and a half? I could cook and serve, but she could feed James, and while he ate, I could stay upstairs for my own meal. The next day Martha said she'd consult with her husband. She reported back: they are remodeling their house, and the extra money would be welcome. She would remain until 6:30 p.m.

Transformation! Now I no longer dread the end of the afternoon. I eat a very early supper, when James does, but by myself, reading the paper or browsing through a magazine. My stomach doesn't clench anymore as James refuses this or that. I am still able to tuck him into bed and sit nearby as he goes to sleep. Thanks for my idea! Thanks for my letting go! Thanks for Martha!

Now I was on a roll. I remembered that I'd had two quiet hours before my night aide came at 10:30 p.m. I had been able to watch a whole episode of *Doc Martin,* an eccentric, funny, and tender series from the BBC. Tom and Ingrid, friends in Seattle, had highly recommended this. (Thank you, BBC! Thank you, Tom and Ingrid!) Then I still had time to read for an hour in *The Girl Who Played with Fire,* second in Stieg Larsson's angry and engrossing trilogy. Thanks for books! Forever and always, thanks for books.

Tomorrow I could go to the gym with my new swimsuit and swim! Exercise! Thank you, thank you. As I finally tuned into the surf of my bedside white-noise machine and began to fall asleep, I actually felt quite cheerful. When was the last time I went to sleep feeling cheerful?

It did not escape my notice that while my thank-yous included a new battery, fish soup, a freezer, a TV show, and a swimsuit, they also made mention of people: Tony, Kim, Martha, and Tom and Ingrid. I knew I could think of more. As I drifted into sleep, I noted that perhaps, after all, I had something that resembled a net.

Since that night, I have tried to maintain this bedtime ritual. I think it has definitely helped. Some nights are easier than others. A few days ago, after a long session in my dentist's chair preparing for a new crown, I was so tired I almost forgot. But then I thought: "Novocaine! I am thankful for novocaine!" I have even learned to be thankful for what *didn't* happen. I didn't faint in the dentist's chair. (I never have, but that doesn't mean I won't.) I don't have to go back to the dentist for three more weeks. Three whole weeks!

I still grit my teeth when someone tells me, with infuriating sanctimony, "Count your blessings!" But I don't produce my practiced phony smile. Instead I reply, "Yes, I do."

AN UNEXPECTED
CORNER OF MY NET

March 10

This is a story about a car that didn't blow up. But it is also a postscript about my net, the web of support all caregivers need. Yesterday I discovered an unexpected corner of my own net in a suburban high school parking lot.

I am not a natural optimist. After my father died when I was seven, I learned how mortal disasters strike without warning. I worry a lot. At any sign of difficulty, I can easily think of all possible catastrophic possibilities. In my late twenties, when I consulted a counselor about my failing first marriage, he once sighed and said, "Susan, instead of just getting on your train, you are always too busy adding a long line of what-if boxcars."

Over the years, however, I've seen that my truth is a little more complicated. I'm not just adding what-ifs. I am often standing on the curb, looking both ways, watching for the train (or bus or runaway car) to appear out of nowhere and knock me down. What I've learned is, of course, that when the blow does finally fall, it never comes from the direction I'm watching. It sneaks up from behind.

Consider James's long battle with Parkinson's and dementia. Although James was fifteen years older than I, when we married he was always so energetic and vigorous—in fact, I often wore out before he did—that I never imagined he would succumb to a long, lingering, debilitating disease. Instead, despite the fact that he had been in excellent health for years and exercised daily, I worried he would have a heart attack or a devastating stroke and die instantly. I worried when he was late coming home in case he had been in an accident. I panicked when he mentioned a pain in his chest (a cracked rib) or dizziness (an inner-ear infection) or stomach trouble (diverticulitis). I always imagined he would die one day at a very old age, seated at his architect's desk, his pencil in his hand as he was making one final, spirited sketch.

James didn't worry like me. We were a salutary balance, since he was sure everything was going to turn out all right, and I was almost equally sure it probably wouldn't. When we traveled together, I would say, "Now we're two hours behind schedule! Our plane will never make the connection!" James would say calmly, "We'll probably make up time. And besides, we can run to the next gate." Meanwhile I would begin to plan ahead, just in case.

Sometimes he was right. We made the next flight. Sometimes I was right. We missed it, but I usually had an idea already in place. Once, landing in a small airport in Scotland, we discovered that friends we were going to meet there had missed their own plane from London. I had suspected that might possibly happen. (Naturally. Even though they were always punctual.) So I could say, "Okay, hon, I've already looked on the map and discovered a park just a few miles from here. Let's eat a sandwich in the airport café, rent a car, and spend the afternoon walking around the park and its gardens until the Coopers arrive." So we did.

In the last few years, I have understood that my relentless planning is part of what makes my net hold together. I have stopped thinking of it as a character flaw. But yesterday I had no plan, no idea. I had to fall back on the unknown. My net.

Early in the morning I left our house for the two-hour drive to our Wisconsin retreat. I've managed to do this several times in the last year, and I believe these brief breaks have helped keep me from plunging over the cliff. I hoped to arrive by noon and have almost forty-eight hours of quiet (interrupted only by phone calls and checks on James, who will always have an aide nearby).

Although our car is ten years old, Tony, our mechanic, keeps it tuned, fit, and running. I was not expecting trouble. For the first time in five months, my planned break did not coincide with a forecast of snow, sleet, or rain turning to ice. The highways were clear.

Forty minutes from our house, I was zooming along with the rest of the high-speed traffic somewhere in open country, listening to Johnny Cash's last recording, just released, mostly songs about death, dying, and trusting in salvation. His weary and gravelly voice brought me comfort.

Then all at once I heard a strange noise in the car. Although I am distressingly ignorant about motors, cylinders, and the innards of automobiles, I can diagnose quite a few noises. I can hear a flat tire (flap, splat), a bad muffler (phut, PHAT), scratchy brakes (screech!), and more. But I hadn't heard this noise before. It was a whistling whoosh, like wind blowing through the car. I thought it came from under the hood, but I wasn't sure.

I quickly checked my windows. All closed. (This is March.) I looked up at the sunroof. I've never liked sunroofs, and I hadn't opened this one for years. Its cover was tightly shut. Doors? Quick glance. Nope. Trunk lid? Not possible. I looked out the windows. Had a gale-force wind just swept over the midwestern prairie? Not a tree was moving. The noise calmed down when I slowed, then amplified again when I speeded up. It easily drowned out Johnny Cash.

So I had to get off the freeway as soon as possible and find out what was wrong. Was something about to break off and explode? I had no idea where I could find a mechanic or even a gas station, since this freeway bypasses the smaller, far-out suburban communities that have slowly spread from the city. All I could see were frozen fields, farms, and more freeway ahead.

I passed one or two exits that didn't promise anything except "210th Street" or "Concord Boulevard." Those signs told me nothing. Then I saw an exit that indicated a community college. Off I turned, hoping that the college might be located in a settlement with a mechanic, not just acres of lonely campus.

The community college was miles from the turnoff. I saw some residential streets here and there, a factory, a large office complex. No gas stations. No stores. More rural land. I wasn't sure which streets to follow. I made random decisions, trying to find a commercial center or indeed anywhere I could stop and ask for help.

Down one road, I abruptly came upon a huge, rambling high school, its parking lot jammed with hundreds of empty vehicles. Here at least I could pull over, get out of the car, and try to locate a possible source of my problem. As I carefully turned into the lot, I noticed a large, old, slightly rusted sedan parked in a spot just above the lot. A very hefty man—late fifties? sixties?—was sitting behind the wheel. He was just sitting there, not doing anything, looking at the parking lot.

I ignored him and stopped my car. I walked around it and examined it carefully. Nothing. I walked across the lot to the front door of the high school. It was locked. I walked back.

Then I looked at the man in his car. Ordinarily I would not walk up to a strange man who was staring at a school parking lot and ask for help. I'm not sure why I decided this was the right thing to do. But I did.

As I stepped bravely toward his car, the man started his motor and rolled down the slope toward me. He opened his window. "I have a problem," I said. "Something is wrong with my car, and I don't know what to do. I'm forty minutes from home, I really don't know exactly where I am, and I have no idea where to find a garage." The man slowly extricated himself from his car. He was very large.

"What's the problem?" he asked, following me toward my parked car. I explained. He too checked the windows, the doors, the trunk. He too was puzzled. "Oh, and I should introduce my-self," I said politely. "My name is Susan Toth." "And I'm Mac," he said after a moment. "I'm the security guard for the parking lot here."

Soon Mac had miraculously squeezed himself into my car, while I sat in the passenger seat, and we went for a test ride. I thought how weird this was: I was heading into who-knows-where with a stranger at the wheel. But I felt relieved. I was no longer alone with my problem. We chatted a little. Mac explained that the high school issued paid permits for parking, and it was his job to make sure no one sneaked in free, not to mention sneak-ing out of school itself.

As soon as we found a stretch of open highway, Mac revved my car up to speed. The whoosh blasted through the car. "Wow!" he said. "I've never heard anything like that." He fiddled with my air-intake control. "Maybe that's it," he said hopefully. For a few minutes we both thought it was. But no.

"So what do I do now?" I asked pitifully. I envisioned myself marooned here, over an hour's drive from our cottage and nearly as far from home. Was my break already ruined before it started? Who would make repairs? How long would this take? How would I get home?

"Tell you what," Mac said, interrupting my catastrophe plan-ning. "I know a great mechanic. I go there myself. He's really good. It's a small shop, only a few miles away. Now, this is how you get there—" He stopped. "You know what?" he continued. "Why don't you follow me in your car, and I can lead you there."

So Mac, willing to leave his post to help me, guided me on a circuitous route (I never would have figured it out), down one road, then another, onto a small side street and right to the door of Specialist Mechanics. He even insisted on getting out of his car again and taking me personally into the shop, where he intro-duced me to the young man behind the counter. "This is Tom," he said. "He'll take care of you. And now I have to get back to work."

I gave Mac a big hug. "You have been my knight in shining armor today, Mac," I said truthfully. I was no longer worried. I was sure Tom would indeed take care of me.

And he did. When his coworker, Steve, returned from a call, he sent Steve with me on another test ride. Moments after the *whoosh* began, Steve had an answer.

"Your sunroof," he said decisively. "Turn right at the next light and pull over." I did. He reached up, slid the cover back, opened the sunroof, and closed it.

"That's it," he said. "The seal just wasn't tight."

"But Steve," I said, almost unable to believe that the solution was so easy, "how could that have happened? I haven't opened the sunroof for years."

"Don't know," he said. "But that's what it is." He was right. The car was blissfully quiet as we drove back to the shop.

No charge. I hugged Steve too. I was so happy that I could continue on my break that I wanted to hug Tom, but he was busy inside. An hour later I was at our cottage, unpacking my groceries, computer, and the third volume of my mystery series.

Last night, as I was slipping into bed, nestled in the quiet of the woods, still savoring gratitude for my safe arrival, for a quiet afternoon and evening, for Mac and Tom and Steve, I pictured a small corner of a large web, rather like one spun by an industrious spider. The web was thin, almost invisible, and surprisingly sturdy. It was my net.

I don't really expect to become an optimist. But yesterday, my net was there.

THE LONG PASSAGE

March 24

> *When I wrote this, the end seemed very near. Months,*
> *not weeks, lay ahead.*

I remember another tunnel.

Almost fifty years ago, when I was a summer-school student in London, I discovered the beauty of ballet. Clutching a standing room ticket on the uppermost tier of the Royal Opera House in Covent Garden, I was enthralled by the dancers of *Swan Lake* floating far below. Although I could not see their faces, I could hear every note of Tchaikovsky's haunting music.

When I left that night, I was in a trance. I descended into the Underground and turned into a dimly lit tunnel that seemed deserted. I was alone, but I was not in the least afraid. Then I heard a faint strain of music, gradually growing stronger as I walked farther. Rounding a corner, I saw a man standing next to the wall and holding a violin. An upturned hat on the pavement held a few scattered shillings. He looked away, somewhere in the distance, as he played, with piercing tenderness, the recurring theme from *Swan Lake*.

As I continued down that darkened tunnel, the music seemed to follow me. It filled the passage like a message, a moment of remembering, until it gradually died away into a whisper and disappeared entirely when I reached the platform where I would wait for the next train. But I kept hearing it, wafting through my mind, all the way back through the London summer night to my well-lit dormitory room.

During the past ten days, I have been thinking about that night. I remember how the melody echoed in the London Underground. I am in a dimly lit passage now, and oh, how I wish I could hear an echo of that music.

Last week, after a particularly difficult night, James fell into an almost unshakable sleep. He slept day and night for almost four days. Each day he awoke briefly—or my aide and I woke him—for a little nourishment, a drink of water, using the bedside commode. But then all he wanted was to go back to sleep. He slept with his mouth open, breathing heavily and steadily.

Mary, our trusted and empathetic hospice nurse, came to visit. "This is a significant change," she said. "He even looks different."

After four days, James woke up. Since then, he has slept very little during the day. He naps for short periods. Some days he will watch a little television or pore over a page from a magazine. He may lie quietly and listen to music. He talks a little. Other days he wants to get out of bed and then in again, because he doesn't know what to do. If he is agitated at night, he gets a small dose of Ativan. Over the past year, he has had brief episodes of dementia when he wonders where home is. One night he cried out in distress, "I want to go home! Why can't I go home?" I find this cry excruciating.

"Weeks," said Mary on her last visit. "Not months, no, no. Weeks."

But of course she doesn't really know. Parkinson's is a cunning beast, and James's will to live is extraordinary. So we are walking through a dark passage, like that Underground tunnel. It twists and turns, and I have no idea how long it is. Everything about dying is mysterious to me.

During each day, I send James's aide upstairs and sit by his bed for a while. I reminisce about this or that or describe how I've just been swimming or walking or grocery shopping. If he is half-asleep and peaceful, I stroke his forehead and try to speak carefully chosen words of comfort. Sometimes he will bring out a single word in reply, hoarse, coming from a great distance. James does not want to talk about dying, even now, and I respect his decision.

So I tell him how much I love him and what our life together has meant to me. I feel no urgency about this, because he has heard it all before, again and again. Thirteen years ago, just before Christmas, James and I landed together in a hospital. It was a freakish and awful coincidence. We had returned a few days before from two chilly if wonderful weeks in London. Both of us brought back nasty colds. Mine morphed into an intense sore throat, so severe that I could hardly swallow. James had a feverish head cold, stuffy nose, and nearly smothered breathing. (A heavy snorer, James also had chronic sleep apnea, something we did not learn until too late.)

Despite his illness, James insisted on attending an important interview for an exciting architectural project. (He didn't get the job.) Then, a day later and even sicker, he was determined to make a brief appearance at the annual Christmas party hosted by our doctor, Eben, and his partner. I stayed in bed. I remember stirring briefly when James returned later in the evening and then falling back into sleep.

When I stumbled out of bed the next morning, James was already downstairs at the dining table. My throat was now so constricted I knew I had to get to an emergency room. When I walked into the dining room, I told James what was happening. "I feel weird too," James said very slowly. "I woke up feeling funny." His words sounded a little slurred. I looked at him closely. His mouth was slightly twisted downward on one side.

"James," I said after a moment, only half-believing, "I think you've had a stroke."

"Oh, my God," he said. "That's all I need." We stared at each other. He followed me up to the bathroom on our landing, and I pointed at his twisted mouth in the mirror.

"We'll have to drive to the emergency room right away," I said. (Did I think of calling 911? No. I reasoned that we were walking, we were talking, we were not in imminent danger. What did I actually know about strokes? Very little. About sleep apnea and its connection to strokes? Nothing.)

Then my daughter woke up. Jenny had heard us talking. As we began fumbling for our clothes, she said, "For heaven's sakes, you can't drive. I'll take you." So she did. The hospital was twenty minutes away.

When we arrived at the emergency room, I walked up to the reception window and said, "I need to see a doctor because my throat is closing up, but I think my husband has had a stroke." I sounded conversational. (In retrospect, I see this as a bit of insanity from a blackly comic sketch.) Within an hour, we were both hospitalized.

I had to fight for the right to be in a bed next to James. Today, with tighter restrictions, we would probably be forced into separate wards, one for infectious disease, one for strokes. I was undoubtedly wrong, but I won.

Once we were both hooked up to IVs, I began to think about strokes. I remembered reading somewhere that a second, much more serious stroke often followed a first, milder one. What if James died during the night? What did I need to tell him?

So I slipped past the flimsy curtain dividing our beds, and I sat on the edge of his. That night I made sure I told James, at length, with lots of repetition, how I felt about him. He joked a little, saying "Enough! Enough!" But I thought of everything possible that needed—and probably didn't need—to be said, and I said it.

Though he did not have another stroke, that turned out to be the beginning of his Parkinson's. In the intervening years, we both have continued to remind each other how blessed we have been in this marriage. Nothing more needs to be said now.

Still, I do keep saying it. I talk in metaphors. I tell James that I am the captain of our ship, and I am sailing with him to a farther shore. I may not be a great navigator, I say, but this is my task, and I am doing my best. It is a mysterious shore ahead, I go on, but because he has known so much love in his life—and has given love in return—I assure him he will continue to know love. I even describe whom he'll see on that shore, as I name parents and friends who have gone before him. Sometimes when I mention a particular name, I'll see a ghost of a smile on his face. "But you probably won't have to see Adelaide," I add, conjuring up an image of his formidable ex-mother-in-law. "No, I don't guess Adelaide will be waiting for you. Of course, maybe she has been utterly transformed. Who knows?" Then he really smiles.

I add that I can't get off the ship myself right now, but when I do arrive, I expect him to be waiting for me with open arms. If he is not too sunk in sleep, James will make a sweeping gesture with his arms, as if describing a hug. "Are you going to be there?" I demand.

"Of course," he whispers.

I told a friend about this metaphor, and she rolled her eyes. Too preachy. Too literal. Too—well, she didn't actually say this, but I got it—too smarmy. But James doesn't think it is smarmy. I told him my ship story again just a few hours ago, and when I was finished, he whispered a single word: "Great!"

And what does my friend know? No more than I do.

Besides, James wants to believe in the continuation of love. Before I met him, he became a very liberal Catholic, free of dogma, utterly uninterested in the Vatican, but committed to the root of faith. (Yes, I understand that many Catholics would say that those qualifiers mean he isn't a Catholic at all. However, he would—and did—serenely shrug off their protests.)

Tomorrow I will get up, make James a little French toast and juice—he is still eating and drinking, just small amounts—and, after my aide comes, work a while at my desk. This morning I started to fill out our census form. It arrived several days ago. But I had to stop almost as soon as I had begun.

The first question asks: "How many people were living or staying in this house, apartment, or mobile home on April 1?" Today is March 24. I can't answer yet.

CENSUS DAY

April 6

Census Day has come and gone. On April 1, I could certify that
two people—James and I—still lived together at one address.
As our ship has drawn ever closer to the far shore, I think James
has decided he is not yet ready to disembark. I imagine his taking
a very deep breath, blowing into our sails, and turning our vessel
aside, back into choppy waters. I have again pulled out my maps
of survival so I can continue to chart our unpredictable course.

LIVING IN A BUBBLE

April 28

My friend Marnie was exasperated. Marnie, who lives in a comfortable Connecticut enclave, had just finished reading these essays and called with a sharp reaction. "You live in a bubble!" she said, and from her admonishing tone, I could sense this was my fault.

"You seem so alone. That's what I just don't get," she went on. "In my neighborhood, we form rotations for anyone who needs help. Why, right now I'm one of a group bringing meals and visits to a seven-year-old boy who is dying of cancer. Where are your friends and neighbors? Where is family?"

Ah. Friends. Neighbors. Family. Although in the last few months, I have identified a network of support, it isn't always there.

Loving and sustaining as they are, my friends can't exactly camp outside my door. One, for example, has been living for months through difficult and time-consuming personal and professional crises. She rushes from one burden to another, trying to keep her own life from overwhelming her. Another travels so often, both for work and family needs, that we mostly catch up with phone calls and very occasional lunches. One encourages me from a thousand miles away. Still another lives so far away that she would have to fly over an ocean to get here.

Not long ago I read, with both sympathy and a sense of fore-boding, a newspaper column by a well-known writer who had recently been widowed. Helping her endure her loneliness, she said, was "a large circle of dear friends." I marveled wistfully at the linking of "dear" and "large circle." As I tried to picture my own friends, all joined together, I left out the casual, let's-have-lunch-sometime, see-you-after-the-ice-melts ones. I concentrated on "dear," friends so close that they always know what is happening to me. My circle was quite small.

Even though I am mostly an introvert, someone who needs quiet time by herself, I wonder how even the most gregarious and outgoing caregivers can keep up "a large circle of dear friends." Where do they find the time? Friendships take maintenance. A full-time caregiver does not have much time-absorbing attention to spread around.

Marnie's neighbors sound exceptional to me. Years ago, I might have shared her assumptions. In the small town where I grew up, many of my widowed mother's friends lived near her. Since she had to teach full-time, she was unable to join in the neighborhood coffee klatches. But she always had a few cherished friends within blocks. Others lived minutes away by car. They could visit easily back and forth.

In my city neighborhood, most people are gone during the day. We do not share churches, PTA, bridge clubs, or morning coffee. We all move in separate orbits. Without children to link us to other families, I never see them.

Not long ago, a woman on our block who is indeed a valued friend—but in her eighties and kept very occupied with her active husband—called me in some anxiety. "Herb and I heard a siren and noticed an emergency vehicle that stopped across the street from your house today. I was so worried it was for James." No, I assured her, it wasn't for us. I had no idea who had been in trouble. I still don't know. Two for-sale signs went up on our block this winter; then they were removed. I never met either the families (or couples, or not) who moved out or moved in. This is not that kind of neighborhood.

A fragment of my net does occasionally pop up even here. The day before last Thanksgiving, as I was walking down the sidewalk, the young mother who lives next door stepped outside and called to me. On the rare occasions we see each other, Elspeth and I exchange friendly greetings, and she knows that James has been ill for a long time. "Would you like some leftovers tomorrow afternoon?" Elspeth asked. "I'll be cooking much more than we can eat."

"I would be thrilled!" I told her, which was true. Caregivers do not have time to stuff and roast turkeys, never mind pureeing squash, sautéing vegetables, or baking pies.

Elspeth's young daughter, then in second grade, arrived the next afternoon proudly carrying a heavy tray. It held a feast of so many delicious courses (I can still remember her airy sweet potato pudding!) that I knew Elspeth, who, like her husband, works very long hours during the week, had spent even longer hours in her kitchen. On this Thanksgiving, I indeed gave thanks. We continued to feast for several days on Elspeth's bounty.

Ever since, Elspeth has remembered us whenever a holiday has given her time to cook. I do not forget to tell her how appreciative I am. Elspeth, however, is an exception in our neighborhood.

With her usual take-no-prisoners honesty, Marnie went on to suggest that my caregiver's loneliness was partly self-inflicted. Since James and I had traveled so often during our years together, perhaps I had failed to make wide-enough connections. "All the couples I know usually take trips with other couples," she said. "You two traveled alone. That always seemed strange to me." She was right. We traveled in a pod of two. Was I now paying an unforeseen price for such a companionable marriage?

Marnie, I reassured myself later, had never been a long-term caregiver. Forming a steady, reliable rotation of caring volunteers in any community is probably easier when the person who is ill is relatively young, mentally acute, and suffering from a disease that will not last for many years. How long can even the most devoted friends and neighbors continue to volunteer their time? Wouldn't they begin to flag? Tire of making and delivering casseroles? Squeezing visits into their crowded lives, week after week, month after month after month? Year after year?

In a way, though, Marnie is right. Many long-term caregivers do live in a bubble. For twenty-four hours a day, a caregiver can never turn away from the ultimate responsibility for the health and life of a person he or she loves.

Even when taking a break, I trail that bubble behind me, sometimes on a long enough string that it can float into the distance, like a kite, almost invisible. But I listen for any phone call—my mobile is always in my pocket—that will instantly make me yank on the string, reel it in, and head home.

Sometimes that bubble is as tough as reinforced glass. On some days an aide has to call in sick or report an emergency that will prevent her from coming. Friends, willing as they might be, cannot be asked to stay with James. Neither he nor I would want them to spoon-feed him a meal or help him to the bathroom. When I am literally unable to leave the house, I feel the windows of our house forming a bubble, reminding me I can't set foot outside our door.

Thankfully, my bubble is not impermeable. Technology has tossed out lifelines. When I was young, long-distance calls were so expensive that my mother kept a three-minute egg timer by the telephone. When the sands ran through its tiny hourglass, the call had to end. Now, for a few cents a minute, I can talk to anyone for hours (except I don't have hours). I can grab my phone, dial, and either hear a familiar, concerned voice, or leave a message, in varying degrees of desperation: "Call back when you have time," or "Please call as soon as you possibly can!"

Sometimes I can almost feel the hugs humming through cyberspace. Yesterday, on a sunny spring morning, I walked for almost an hour around our nearby lake. As soon as I left our house, I called a cherished friend whom I haven't seen for almost three years. Before she moved far away, ten years or more ago, we taught together, raised our single children (both dramatic daughters), and found ourselves in unexpected and happy second marriages. We know a lot about each other.

When I started my walk, I had slowly been sinking for days into a slough of sadness, a boggy hollow that can turn into a quicksand of hopelessness, sucking me deeper and deeper. When Julie answered, I found my footing again. I talked, she listened. I complained, she commiserated. She didn't try to cheer me up. Instead she said things like "How awful!" or "I can't believe it!" or "No wonder!" I soaked in empathy like a dry sponge.

At home, with James and my aides, I try to be steady, smiling, and positive. James's children don't call in order to hear my woes. My own daughter doesn't like to read these essays. She loves me, and they depress her. So I need my friends to hear me out, understand, and respond. Somehow I always seem to know which number to dial.

I also depend for support on e-mails. Although the Internet can overburden us with information, it is a lifesaver for caregivers. E-mails from my friends zoom like little bolts of reassuring light into my bubble. Some write more, others less. (It is not a medium everyone likes.) One couple sends me their mutual reviews of movies I might like—or I should avoid. Another forwards jokes that sometimes I skim and delete, but occasionally I snort with laughter. One correspondent I've yet to meet—we connected through one of my books—sends me assorted clippings, mostly about travel in Britain, from the *Washington Post*. Since I am a writer and a very fast typist, I "talk" in an e-mail as naturally as I talk on the phone. I never know when I'll be free to have a real-time conversation, so I value the ability to read an e-mail and reply when I can. My friends know why my answers are often very short.

So far I have avoided Internet forums and chat rooms. I know they offer great solace to many caregivers. But I lack the desire, time, and emotional energy such continuing participation requires. I don't want to plunge into roundtable conversations in cyberspace.

What I have instead is a small but essential resource of five women who have been caregivers for their husbands. Four of those husbands died in the recent and not-so-recent past. One has a husband who has long been in a nursing home, but she still faithfully visits and tends him there. Two are old friends of mine, and I met the other three through mutual acquaintances. We differ in age from fifty to eighty-plus. Not one of them knows any of the others. We are not a group, but singly they encourage and support me in ways no one else can.

Barb, the youngest, was married, like me, to an older man with Parkinson's and dementia, and she cared for him at home until the end. Still on the rise in a demanding profession and scheduled almost to the minute, she makes time for me whenever I need encouragement. "Whatever you're doing is right," she says, again and again. Unlike most of my (noncaregiving) friends, she has never urged me to place James in a nursing home. "You can do this," she repeats. "You will be glad later that you did." When I confess my lapses, she says emphatically, "You are doing a great job. Yes, you are! You are doing a great job!"

When Barb and I meet for an occasional snatched hour in a coffee shop, we understand each other. She knows why I wonder if I can go on. We also laugh a lot. Dumb decisions? Close escapes? Well-meaning but tactless remarks? We can match stories.

Those whose husbands have died can also advise me, gently and lovingly, about what lies ahead. After I told Barb last month that our hospice nurse and I both (wrongly) thought James had only weeks to live, she paused, put down her coffee cup, and said, "Susan, I've wanted to wait for the right time to tell you this. Now is the time."

She reached across the coffee-shop table and took my hand. Holding my gaze, she said, "This is hard to hear, but you need to hear it. When James dies, you don't have to call the hospice team right away. Say your good-byes first. Give yourself as much time as you need. Then don't tell the funeral home to come to your house immediately. You may not be ready. You'll know."

"Okay," I said.

"But here is what you really need to know," Barb went on. "Don't be in his room when the men from the funeral home arrive. You don't want to see them zip up the body bag."

This may have been the most important piece of practical advice I received at the end. Who else but another caregiver could have told me that? A picture flashed into my mind. I knew instantly Barb was right.

"Call a friend," she added. "Someone you really trust. Then wait with her upstairs. Maybe you'll want to walk out to the van with the attendants. Maybe not. Later I wished I had. It was senseless guilt, but still . . ."

These five caregiver friends all know I am writing these essays. Three of them had married men with children from a first marriage. Not long ago one of these former stepmothers said, "When are you going to write about stepchildren? Are you going to tell our stories? Caregiving as a stepmother?"

Marnie had asked me in disbelief, "So where is family?" My friend was right. I do need to write briefly about caregivers and stepchildren. My own immediate family of origin is quite small. I have one married sister, who has two grown daughters, and I have one daughter. Although an affectionate clan, sympathetic to each other's vagaries, we all live far apart: California, North Carolina, New York, Virginia. Like most of my closest friends, they cannot rush to my door on a moment's notice. Yet I can quickly reach them by phone or e-mail. So, Marnie, where is family? Here, but not here. Certainly not baking casseroles, running errands, or trying to take care of James. But here, just the same.

I also have six adult stepchildren. Four live in town, and the other two keep in touch from distant states. All of James's children have held him close to their hearts. When our Parkinson's specialist told us a year ago, "Now is the time for family to take care of unfinished business," I could tell her honestly that they had no need of deathbed reconciliations.

Early in his disease, while he was still able to leave the house, James's local children went out with him to lunch or to a movie. They sometimes came over to our house to watch a football game or a DVD with their father while I ran errands. During the past two years, as James's condition worsened and he could no longer leave the house for excursions, they have helped in many ways, from sleepovers to bringing him homemade treats. The out-of-towners visit when they can, and even though he can no longer respond with more than a word to a telephone, they call so he can hear their voices.

But, like my friends, their lives are already crammed with full-time jobs, family obligations, and social life. All are married with children. They have in-laws as well, who, in varying degrees of health, need attention. How could I possibly expect them to set aside regular hours from their weekends, the only time they have to spend with their own families, do their shopping or laundry or cleaning, and try to keep up their friendships?

My little group of stepmother-caregivers agree that we must all tread carefully. "Number one rule for a stepmother," one of my friends said tersely, "is, Keep your mouth shut." We know we cannot inquire, probe, or criticize. I can say to my own daughter, "Are you really going to wear those tight jeans?" or "How did you ever get yourself into that mess?" or "I'm really upset about what you said this morning. Do you know how that sounded?" She can answer back, offer her own (sometimes equally unwelcome) criticisms, and depend on our mutual love and respect to see us through a tangled thicket.

So a stepmother can ask for help, within limits, but she has to accept refusal graciously. Her own needs may be ignored. She cannot complain. Even one harsh word to a stepchild can sour a relationship. During a parent's long illness, especially toward the end, emotions run high. Children may feel they need to reclaim their father. Sometimes funerals hold added grief because a stepmother can learn unpleasant truths about her resented place in her husband's family.

"We were married for fifteen years," Dolores told me, "and Charlie had been divorced for ten years before that. We almost never saw his two boys. They both lived in Boston. High-powered careers. They stayed away during his radiation and chemo treatments. But when Charlie lapsed into his final coma, they came to town ready to arrange his funeral. One was so sure he knew what was right that he wanted to cancel the plans Charlie and I had worked out together. They also wanted a more elaborate and expensive reception—which they naturally assumed I'd pay for. I was so vulnerable. I broke down and wept, and we barely spoke after the funeral."

"I think Greg's kids never got over the idea that he had remarried," said another friend. "So when he was dying, I had to face the fact that all my years as what I thought was a loving stepmother simply didn't count. It was really weird. They acted as if I weren't there—no, I take that back, they acted as if I were a wood post uncomfortably stuck in their way—and they brushed right by me. I guess they were so caught up in their own grief that they couldn't pay any attention to what I was feeling. Greg used to say that if something ever happened to him, his kids would be there for me. He was so positive. I knew differently, and I'm sorry to say I was right."

In their retirement Len and Pat had taken to travel with zest. During their twenty years together, they often returned to Paris, their favorite city, for two-week visits, and they gradually explored other parts of Europe, Africa, and the Far East. Meanwhile, during those same years, Len's children were raising their own young families. "When Len's MS got bad, his girls kept their distance," Pat reported. "Did they offer to help? Not really. I think they felt that I'd had all the goodies, and now it was payback time. This was my job, and they were going to let me do it."

Another family, not available to every caregiver, has kept me company in my bubble. By now several of my aides have probably spent as much or more accumulated time with me as any of my stepchildren. I see them so often they know most of my quirks, and I knew a few of theirs. I know who is a vegetarian and who likes bittersweet dark chocolate. I understand why someone needs to sleep late, past her shift, and why someone else needs bagels and strong coffee right away in the morning. They have heard stories about my life, and I know a little (or a lot) about their boyfriends or husbands or parents.

Together we have confronted unnerving moments with James—a fall averted, a frightening bout of anxiety, a violently upset stomach, sneezes that won't stop, messy accidents. They have assisted him and me with the most intimate of tasks. I trust them, and that means I can lay down some of my responsibility—not all, but quite a bit—for hours at a time.

My aides know when I am very tired or upset. I tell them. I don't worry, as I do with my stepchildren, that I might sound as if I were whiny about James. My aides understand the toll of minute-by-minute, day-by-day, long-term care. Yes, I pay my aides, but they have responded over months and years with loyalty, tenacity, and affection I could never have expected. They too are family.

I can still sometimes feel unbearably lonely. Despite Marnie's remonstrances, I don't think this is unusual. Because of Parkinson's and its accompanying dementia, I have lost the lively company and conversation of the best friend I have ever had—not just my husband and my lover, but my friend.

If I do live in a bubble, however, I am not trapped there. Its walls expand, and I can reach beyond it. I am not without love, friendship, and support. I plan to stay in this bubble with James until the end.

UNMOORED

May 13

I have become unmoored.

I remember this feeling. Some years ago, I was hired as a very minor lecturer for a five-day trip between New York and London on the old *Queen Elizabeth II,* the only ocean liner that still made regular transatlantic crossings. Although James had sailed across the Atlantic several times (beginning with his service in World War II), I had never been on the water for longer than an eight-hour ferry trip.

So I was thrilled to be asked. James's one-way passage, like mine, would be paid. We would sail away together. From old movies I had absorbed images of romance and glamour on the high seas. What woman my age hadn't seen *An Affair to Remember?* Wrapped in furs or chic trench coats, passengers sat in deck chairs and sipped cocktails or tea. Fog misted around them, waves broke over the bow, the boat sparkled at night as it drove through the dark water.

I had always loved the ocean. Living in the middle of America, I did not get to an ocean often. So when I did, if I found a beach where I could walk at the edge of incoming surf, I could blissfully disappear from time. On a rocky coast, if I could sit for an hour or more and watch white foam break in deafening swirls below me,

I was utterly at peace. Back home, landlocked once again, I would turn my white-noise machine to the mechanical sound of imaginary waves splashing onto an imaginary shore. Now I could listen to the real sound for five days. I would be so happy.

Sadly, I wasn't. By the second day, I was quietly terrified. Partly I was unnerved by the constant vibration of the engine, an unceasing reminder that I was not on solid ground. Below me, not so very far below, was an unknown world of water. That dark water sank down, down, down into depths where humans had never penetrated. Our ship was a speck floating on the surface of all that darkness.

When I looked around me, making my way carefully from one side of the deck to the other, I saw only an endless procession of waves. All the waves looked alike. They were rolling away from us, moving toward a shore somewhere, but that shore was so far away I couldn't envision it. I felt I was looking at infinity.

During those five days, I don't remember even a glimpse of another ship. No tankers. No container ships. Nothing but water. No sign that we were not scarily alone on the ocean.

Over my lifetime, I have often walked away some of my fears and sorrows. I find great comfort in setting a brisk pace around our nearby city lake, an easy circle of almost three miles. I like to walk almost anywhere, even just to our co-op (twenty minutes by foot) or drugstore (less than half an hour), and back home again. On our many trips together, James and I walked miles every day, on city sidewalks, down riverside trails, across meadows and moors. When he was healthy, I don't think many days passed when we didn't walk somewhere together.

Now, on board a ship, I found that we only had one route. We could, and did, walk around and around the promenade deck. Large as the *QEII* was, walking that deck didn't take very long. We would circle once and then circle again. We walked in the morning, and we walked after lunch and dinner. Around and around and around. We weren't going anywhere. We were simply floating. Around and around and around. I felt eerily marooned and a little panicky.

That is exactly how I feel right now.

Six weeks ago, our hospice nurse said, "Weeks, not months." I was filled with grief, my eyes brimming every day, my knees wobbly. My stomach ached. But I also sensed a movement, with an end in sight.

Then James rallied. He has such an ingrained fighting spirit. Even with his quality of life—an indefinable concept—so diminished, even as he has to struggle to wake up in the morning, even as his mental focus slips in and out, even as he can no longer read or engage in any conversation of more than a sentence or two, even as he finds his only entertainment in watching television or DVDs that he may or may not follow, James still intends to live until life is wrenched from him.

A few days ago, Dr. Sutton, our Parkinson's specialist, generously took time to write me a quick e-mail. How was James doing? She hadn't had an update for a few months. I wrote back: he is mostly bedbound, often locked into a confused inner world, unpredictable in his daily patterns. But he still relishes food. Swallowing is becoming a problem, but he takes his time. He eats. He can get out of bed, with help, and he has a grip of iron on his supporting bed pole. Sometimes when I want him to let go and sink back onto the bed, I can barely uncurl his fingers.

Janet wrote back almost immediately. "If he is still eating with enthusiasm, you have several months to go," she said. She does not waste time on banalities or sentimental reassurance.

Months, not weeks. How many? Who knows? We are entering our ninth month of hospice. I am not abandoning ship, but I am unmoored.

THE BASE LINE

May 27

A s I begin to fall asleep, I have learned to avoid thinking ahead, with a reassuring ripple of serenity. "Oh, yes! Martha is coming to help tomorrow after breakfast. I spent today doing all of my errands, and I can put off dealing with taxes another day. So tomorrow I will have a free morning!" My assumption is a mistake. It will alert the caregiver's goblin.

This goblin is the one who makes me trip as I take a carton of blueberries out of the refrigerator. I am hurrying too much, as usual, and I catch my shoe on an edge of the rug. All the blueberries spill over the rug. The rug is not very clean. It is also multicolored, with a dark blue and red intricate pattern that absorbs blueberries into invisibility. Until I step on one, then another. Squish. Splat.

This is the goblin who pokes quite early at my sleeping husband, who ordinarily might not awake until eight, and so, as I start to eat my Cheerios, I see on my video monitor that James is trying to get out of bed. As I start up from the dining table, I jiggle and spill my cup of tea. Splash. Slop.

After I hurry downstairs with James's glass of orange juice, which I hope will let him fall back to sleep for long enough so I can finish my cereal (if not my tea), I tip the glass a little too high.

He can't swallow that much. It dribbles damply down his pajama top. I will need to change that immediately, as well as take time to make him newly clean and dry after a night of unbroken sleep.

Sometime about now, I recognize that the day has already taken on a certain aspect, a definite character, something that threatens to become a metaphor for my life.

I don't put a name to this aspect until after I have returned to my (soggy) cereal. I sink back into my chair and try to eat slowly. I sip at a new cup of tea. But for several days, my digestive system has been antsy. It doesn't like stress. It reacts in different ways. This morning, I feel very bloated and gassy, and fortunately, since I am alone in this room (and except for James downstairs, in the entire house), I can afford to indulge in briefly releasing that gas.

Only, I grasp almost instantaneously, with shock, that wasn't gas.

As I race upstairs, needing to clean up another mess—and the morning has barely begun—I think that this is a day that will be dominated by the now-common four-letter excretory word that the *New York Times* still won't print.

When I finally finish my breakfast, I go down to the basement bedroom to let out my three cats. Three is too many these days. Two is too many. Even one seems a bit much. But I've had them all for ten years, and they are my cats. However, my affection for them drops precipitously when I open the door. They didn't like being kept waiting so long. One (I'll never know which) has again deposited a watery pile on the wood floor. Another (also unidentifiable) has thrown up on the Indian-print bedspread, which has been washed so often it has an antique patina.

Martha arrives. I clean up the cat messes. After fixing James's breakfast and doing the dishes, I go downstairs to help her. For today is Dynamite Day.

Almost all Parkinson's patients suffer from constipation. Early in Parkinson's, mild measures, combined with attention to diet, can help. Later, which is where James is now, every third day—if no action has occurred—a suppository is necessary, so powerful and usually so immediately effective that my caregivers and I call it The Dynamite.

Did I ever imagine that I would be able to deal with The Dynamite? To my surprise, I can. It helps hugely that James not only cooperates but somehow—I think by pretending that all this is not happening—maintains his dignity. I don't know how he does it.

Once absorbed into the body, The Dynamite continues to work, sometimes with unexpected and intermittent explosions over several hours. So cleanup continues too. By early afternoon, I had spent all my free hours so far dealing with one mess or another.

Mess is an inescapable element of caregiving. I've mostly come to terms with the housekeeping muddle—diapers and bed pads stashed here and there, tabletops heaped with salve, creams, lotions, antiseptic wipes, sprays, latex gloves, paper towels, almost enough stuff to stock a small drugstore (see "Stuff, Stuff, Stuff"). I am mostly used to the muddle. But a year ago I didn't have to pay so much attention to this other messiness. Now I do.

Most caregiving manuals I've read glide smoothly, tactfully—and quite quickly—over the personal hygiene topic usually listed in the index as "Toilet." I took good advice from a former caregiving spouse, who is a mother with grown children. She told me, "You know, when my boys were young, I cleaned them up. How long before they were all toilet-trained? It took a while. And then later, when someone got sick to his stomach, who had to deal with stinky goo? Remember all that? Really, you'll find that this is not such a big deal."

She was right. Armed with those latex gloves, a washable (and disposable) cellulose cloth, adult-size wipes, a bowl of warm soapy water, and a determinedly cheerful attitude, I soldier on. I am very matter-of-fact about it all. Hey, I think to myself, if James can handle this, so can I.

My caregiver friends listen with sympathy to tales about my

learning curve. It is a great relief to talk to someone who doesn't wince or flinch when I describe something that would make a noncaregiver run for the front door. We all have our own dramatically comic stories. Why not lighten our burdens by sharing them?

Once, when I was half-laughing, half-moaning about a misjudgment I'd made in early days about use of The Dynamite, Dolores said with wicked glee, "Hey, I can top that! The fall Charlie got sick, I recarpeted our bedroom floor. What was I thinking? Maybe I just decided that after twenty years, I didn't need to look at all those worn spots and stains anymore. The new carpet was such a beautiful light blue. The first time I tried something like your Dynamite on Charlie, I didn't have sense enough to spread a cloth underneath the commode. He didn't make it there in time. I stood there watching as everything poured down." She was colorfully descriptive about "everything."

"So what did you do then?" I asked, leaning forward. (I now keep a cheap plastic tablecloth ready to be spread under the commode in James's room.)

"Well, I took care of Charlie first. When he was finally back in bed, I spent an hour on my hands and knees with a pail of cold water, rags, sponges, Woolite, and old towels. Then I put the rags and towels into a plastic bag and threw it out. Next day I got two different carpet cleaners. Everything eventually came out. Sort of."

"Wow," I said.

"You know," Dolores went on, "you do what has to be done. And isn't that maybe the base line? What it all comes down to? You love someone, so you do what has to be done."

After our call ended, I let my shoulders slump with relief. For a while, the goblin had disappeared. I still had my feet planted on the base line.

VANISHING PERSPECTIVE

June 23

A yellow banana, a flowery mug, and a white plastic shower-head: picture them on my lavender Formica kitchen counter, carefully arranged so that light from the window above casts just the right luminous shadows.

Does this perhaps remind you—if you are a museumgoer—of a Dutch still life? Everyday objects glowing with intensity and color?

For me, this still life is an example of vanishing perspective. I am not thinking of an artist's perspective, which I learned about years ago when I was briefly an art history major. No, this vanishing perspective is mine. Each of these three objects is a reminder to me of how my patience has frayed during these recent months of caregiving.

Now I tend to lose perspective on my life at unpredictable times. I move through many of my days in something of a blur. I know my memory is working more or less fine, since I remember my dental appointments, solve occasional obscure clues in the Sunday crossword, and recall my deceased Aunt Clara's middle name (Otelia), but sometimes I find it hard to remember what happened yesterday. Most days are very much alike, differing perhaps in whether I need to go to the grocery store or not, escape for a bike ride or a walk, empty the garbage, or do another load of laundry.

I recently read an essay about caregiving in the *New York Times Sunday Magazine*. Katy Butler, the writer, cited a 2007 study of the DNA of family caregivers of people with Alzheimer's disease. "The ends of the caregivers' chromosomes, called telomeres," she noted, "had degraded enough to reflect a four-to-eight-year shortening of lifespan." I think I can envision my own telomeres looking like ragged seaweed swaying underwater, their fringed tops ready to break apart with the next turbulent wave. (Will they soon wash ashore and rot?) Maybe my degraded telomeres are causing my loss of perspective.

I need to get it back. That is why I try to picture that banana, mug, and showerhead.

First, the banana.

I could not continue without help, but I have not had my house to myself for three years. Helpers come and go, using my refrigerator (essential if they are staying through lunch), snacking (with my permission) on anything left on the counter, showering, leaving used drinking glasses or toothbrushes here and there. Someone who isn't such a solitude-loving person wouldn't mind much. But me? Sometimes—well, take the banana.

I eat a banana every morning with my Cheerios. Once in a while, I vary my breakfast, but mostly I reach for that banana (and a handful of sliced almonds, plus any berries I've stashed away). A morning banana is essential. When James and I rented vacation apartments or cottages, he understood we'd have to find a supermarket if I was running out of bananas. Maybe we all have our little dependencies. A morning banana is one of mine.

Before my kind stepson Frank leaves after his weekly overnight vigil with his father, he usually fixes himself breakfast. One morning not long ago, I wandered into the kitchen after my own breakfast (I was on duty then, and Frank had slept late), and I saw Frank peeling a banana and popping it into his mouth. Just the day before, I had made a grocery run, and I had carefully calculated how many bananas I'd need for the next four or five days. *Was Frank eating one of those bananas?*

I refrained from comment. He was doing me an immense favor by giving up one night a week. I could surely spare him a banana. But, I thought grumpily, this meant I'd have to go back to the store a day earlier than planned. On a Saturday. I hate shopping on Saturdays.

As Frank prepared to leave for his office, he gathered up his belongings from the front hall. They included satchels of newly washed laundry and several paper bags of groceries. Temporarily living in a rented room (during a divorce), he liked to do a week's worth of cooking in my kitchen and then store his one-dish meals in his office. Kitchen and laundry facilities were little enough for me to provide.

But this morning I was brooding about that banana. Then I saw a bunch of bananas sticking out of one of his grocery bags. "Frank," I said accusingly, pointing at the bag. I still cannot believe I actually said this, but I did, oh, yes, I did: *"You owe me a banana!"* Frank stared at me, understandably puzzled. I explained. I had just returned from grocery shopping, and so on.

"Susan," Frank said gently, "I didn't eat your banana. That was my banana. I just bought these."

Only if I had squashed a ripe banana in my face could I have apologized adequately. Maybe not even then. But as I squirmed, Frank started to laugh. So did I. Thank God for laughter. Also for Frank. So we parted with a hug—and each with our own adequate supplies of bananas.

That was when I knew my perspective had become seriously skewed.

Second, the mug.

About a week later, I had returned in late afternoon from a night at our retreat in the Wisconsin woods. That should have restored my perspective completely. But, I'm sorry to report, it hadn't. After James was in bed that night, and I had unpacked and put away my food, clothes, and books, I sleepily went into the kitchen to set out my dishes for breakfast. (Yes, breakfast again. Breakfast matters.)

I always reach for one particular mug. I like my Earl Grey tea, with milk, in a coffee-style mug rather than a cup. On a rare, slapdash shopping trip to a discount store in a nearby mall, I had recently found the perfect one. It was very large, handsomely patterned with vaguely Mexican flowers, shapely with a stemmed pedestal. It was so capacious that I didn't have to refill it, and I could carry it down to James's room without sloshing tea on the way. I loved drinking my tea from that mug.

I couldn't find my mug on the shelf. I do have other cups and mugs in different sizes and colors. I moved them around, looking behind and between for my mug. Nowhere. I knew I'd left it on the shelf two days ago.

Of course. A helper had used it (fine) and had forgotten to return it to the kitchen. So I quietly crept into James's room and searched everywhere with a very small flashlight. No mug. Maybe someone had brought it down to the laundry room? Downstairs to the basement. Up to the living room. Down to a bathroom. Now I had become possessed. Where was my mug? How could it have disappeared so completely? Up to my computer desk. No. Up and down, rechecking places I'd already looked, thinking of new places, wondering, increasingly irritated. *I wanted my mug!*

When I finally went to bed, having wasted at least half an hour of unredeemable time in my futile search, I was still thinking about that mug.

When Martha arrived the next morning, the first question I asked her was, "Martha, have you by any chance seen a large flowered mug with a stem?"

"Oh, yes," she said brightly. "When I came to replace Trish while you were gone, she had just made herself a pot of coffee.

So I told her to take the biggest cup on the shelf and bring it back next time."

Problem solved. Perspective still out of whack.

Third, the showerhead.

When I take a shower, I like a fine spray, not a steady pulse. Our over-the-tub showerhead is rather difficult to twist from one setting to another, but before my overnight helpers arrived, I never thought about it. The head was always set on spray. Except someone else, I discovered, liked the bam-bam pulse. Not everyone. Sometimes the setting stayed on spray. I couldn't predict when I'd forgetfully step into a shower—I never remembered to check first—and find an uncomfortable pulse beating down on my back. Muttering, I would turn off the shower, detach the shower hose, fiddle with the head, and restart the whole process. Then I forgot about it until the next time.

One night, flattened, already half-asleep, I turned on the shower, got into the tub, and got hit with the pulse. As I turned in the tub, my foot almost slipped on the mat. A new, jagged crack appeared in my perspective.

During the next week, I determinedly tried to pinpoint the culprit. Frank? "I never touch the showerhead!" he protested. Trish? "Certainly not!" One by one, helper by helper, I brought up the subject of showerheads. Only with my last try did I discover that Amy was my Pulse Person. "Yes, that's me," she said immediately. "Is that a problem?" No, I explained sheepishly, not really a problem. It was just that I found it hard to remember, and so on. "Of course I'll always change it back," she said, "now that I know."

I was abashed. My long perspective, and who knows how long, is watching James die, very slowly, millimeters at a time. But my short perspective? Crazy focus on a banana, a mug, a showerhead? If they do constitute a still life, it is probably one that only Salvador Dalí, connoisseur of the strange and disturbing, might have wanted to paint.

FRENCH TOAST

July 4

Suddenly we are at the beginning of the beginning of the end.

I use those stuttering qualifiers because with Parkinson's, no one knows exactly when the end will arrive. In the last few weeks, after a change in his medication (which may or may not have jolted him closer), James has begun showing many classic symptoms of late-stage Parkinson's: rigidity, a masklike face, a disappearing voice that can only whisper occasional words, more difficulty in swallowing, a continuing withdrawal from the world around him. His dementia is not much worse. But he is often looking into the distance as if he sees something there that I do not.

Most significant to me, James is no longer interested in eating. He can only tolerate a few bites of food or sips of liquid, and I don't think he cares much about what is in the spoon. Following our hospice nurse Mary's mantra, "Less is more," my aides and I are no longer attempting the impossible task of putting any pounds on his scarily bony frame. Mary says his body may not need any food. It is probably starting to shut down.

As I look back on these last few years, I see so many changes. One constant has always been James's finicky attention to food. His taste buds became chameleons, but he always liked to eat.

Just yesterday, faded as he is, he opened his mouth widely when he saw three cut-up, fresh, homegrown strawberries. He was too tired to chew the last one. I can no longer comfort him with food. I feel this as another wrenching loss.

Only two weeks ago, I could. One morning I bent over him after he had woken for a late breakfast. His face, not quite as masklike, looked troubled, wrinkles between his brows. "James," I asked apprehensively, "is something wrong? Do you hurt?" He whispered something. I put my ear close to his lips. I asked again, slowly and clearly, "Do you hurt?"

"Yes," he whispered. I was startled. He had never said that before. (Parkinson's is not usually a painful disease. Debilitating, destroying, but not painful.)

"What hurts?" I asked. I strained again to catch his whisper.

"My psyche," he said. Then he closed his eyes.

I did not know what to say. For months, at different times, I have talked to James about the journey we are on, using metaphors he can follow. I think he still understands some of what I say, and sometimes he has been able to reply "That is comforting" or even just "Good." Recently he has no longer been thrashing in nighttime agitation or crying out with fear from unarticulated dreams. He has seemed peaceful. This morning, however, he was not. His spirit was in pain.

I knew he would not be able to find many words to tell me more.

He opened his eyes again and just looked at me.

I so badly wanted to help. I did not think this was the time to launch into another metaphoric journey.

So I said, "Well, darling, I can't probably do much about that." I paused. Then I smiled, a conspiratorial sort of smile he knows well, and added, "But I can fix you my famous French toast."

He almost imperceptibly smiled back. I can never convey

the warmth, the delight, the shared glee, of James's smiles. Even this faint, slight one. If I had not been watching him so closely, I would have missed it. I kissed him and went upstairs to make French toast.

I remember many year ago, when I read Nora Ephron's funny, satisfyingly vengeful novel, *Heartburn,* how she included recipes in her tale about a food writer whose husband is unfaithful. Food and love have always been intertwined. I cannot write any more about death today. So I will add my recipe for Susan's French Toast.

Break two or three large eggs into an oblong bowl, big enough to soak one or more pieces of bread, preferably ciabatta or English muffin bread, anything thick and white. (James doesn't like whole grains.) Add a substantial slosh of half-and-half with a smaller slosh of whipping cream. Whip with a fork. Now add a generous shake of cinnamon (do not stint on the cinnamon!), a noticeable sprinkling of ground cardamom, a dash of almond extract, perhaps another dash of vanilla extract if the mood strikes you, a little salt, and at least one large spoonful of dark Jamaican rum. Use the fork again to blend the mixture. It should smell wonderful. If not, add more cinnamon, cardamom, and definitely more rum.

Soak your slices of spongy white bread in the bowl. Melt oodles of butter in a frying pan over medium to low heat. Before the butter browns, gently transfer the slices of bread (you will need to soak them one or two at a time) into the wavy pond of melted butter. You should see butter oozing from below the bread. When you think one side is probably browned, turn the toast. Very gently. It will be heavy with eggs and cream. You will want to eat it. Unless you are feeling thin, don't.

Serve with a mixture of melted butter and real maple syrup. I heat butter and syrup together in a glass measuring cup in the microwave. Pour over toast. Cut into small pieces for someone who has trouble with utensils. Just for now, watch someone eat it and be happy.

This morning James almost choked on his tiny glass of orange juice, into which I had crushed his medications. I do not think he will eat my French toast again.

During the last few months, as I have written these occasional short essays, I have often wondered, "Will this be the last one?" I never know. When the time comes, I do not plan to keep a journal of grief. I have read too many.

So today I ask myself, "What if my very last entry is titled 'French Toast'? Is this how I would want to conclude a long account of my caregiver's journey?" Then I imagine telling this to James. I can guess how he would react. He would laugh.

FIRESTORM

July 24

*Earlier in my introduction, I wrote about this last
night. Some of these details will be familiar. I cannot
bring myself to edit them out.*

James died on Wednesday, July 7.

After finishing "French Toast," I think I knew. When I pictured James laughing at my story—he had not been able to laugh out loud for a long time—I had a feeling that I would not be writing as a caregiver again.

For the previous week, James had been almost entirely bedbound. He slept throughout the night and off and on throughout the day. He spoke very little. He also seemed to have even more trouble swallowing, though Martha did not think he was much worse. Nor did the gentle, loving, and quietly ecumenical priest, Father Pat, who, though retired, came to see his old parishioner when needed. On the Saturday before James died, I asked Pat to stop in for a little while. I left them alone together.

When Pat departed, he said, "I think he was more alert and focused than when I was here a few weeks ago." Pat did not believe an end was near. Then he urged me to think about taking a short break at our Wisconsin retreat. I must have looked glassy-eyed.

"Maybe," I said doubtfully. Our blufftop cottage is an almost two hours' drive away.

Two days later, on Monday afternoon, Mary came to check on James. She was now doing this twice a week. Like Martha, she did not see or hear any dramatic change. She listened carefully to his lungs. She watched him swallow a little water. Shaking her head, she said, "It is all getting harder for him." But she too suggested I should leave for Wisconsin. Long ago, she had said to me, "It is my job to take care of both of you."

I tried to picture myself turning onto the highway leading out of the city, feeling a gradual disburdening. Not now. I couldn't imagine being that far from home. I must have known, and yet I didn't.

On Tuesday morning, James slept long enough for me to finish breakfast, and then I fed him a little tapioca pudding. When Martha arrived, I told her I was going for a half-hour swim at an outdoor pool and then a brief stop at a grocery store. I would be back in two hours. Except in the pool, I would have my cell phone in my pocket. As I left, Martha had James propped up in the bed.

When I returned, I came downstairs to James's room, as I always did when I'd been out of the house. He had just fallen asleep. He looked flushed. I touched his face softly. "I think he has a fever," I said uneasily to Martha. The thermometer told me that, yes, James's temperature had risen slightly. In an hour, it zoomed to 100.5°F. I could hear gurgling as he breathed, not a new sound, but not one that usually lasted very long. This was different. "I want to call Mary right now," I said.

The rest of the afternoon is a blur. Mary was delayed—another patient had unexpectedly died—and Martha and I took turns sitting by James's bed. Most of the time his eyes were closed. He was panting, as if he were running a marathon. When I sat next to him, holding his hand and stroking his face, I talked a little. I didn't need to say much. I had said everything that needed saying many, many times. Sometimes he opened his eyes, and although he looked at me, I do not think he saw me. He was working very hard at breathing.

Around 5:00 p.m., Mary hurried into the room. I had also phoned one of James's daughters, who had been involved in his care, and now Anne sat quietly in the room. With just a brief examination, Mary knew what was happening. She ordered morphine, atropine, and Ativan, and she carefully wrote out for me what to give, when, and how. I called another aide to stay with me during the evening after Martha left. Anne called her five siblings. One got the call at her office in New York City, left immediately with only her purse, took a taxi to the airport, and got on the next available plane to Minneapolis. She arrived after midnight, just in time.

When Mary left, she warned me, "Get some rest. This could go on for days. It could go on for a week. Or it could be sooner."

It was sooner. By 2:00 a.m., James was gone.

He had died at home. That was what I had wanted.

I can't write any more about that night, or the predawn hours afterward, or the arrival of the van from the funeral home. I did what had to be done. I got through it.

After a memorial service several days later, then interment of James's ashes in a beautiful lakeside plot, my caregiver's task was over.

Two weeks later, people ask me, "How are you doing?" I don't know what to say. Any long-term caregiver for someone with a chronic, progressive disease with dementia probably struggles with warring emotions. The battleground is constantly shifting. Numbness, disbelief, stabbing pain, relief, anxiety, calm, guilt, satisfaction, unnerving questions, blankness. A gradual sense of slowing down. Less whirring. Brief peace. Then stabbing pain again. A return of numbness.

I usually answer, "I think I'm doing okay." What else can I say?

A RING AMONG THE ASHES

A Year Later

S ometimes, when I am far from home, I take comfort in pictur-
ing James's wedding ring.

When James and I decided to get married, he designed two
matching wedding rings. Carrying a simple sketch, he happily
marched me into a goldsmith's shop. Both rings would be broad
gold bands, with a hexagonal raised surface in the center. On my
ring, as if it were a tiny canvas, James instructed the goldsmith to
inscribe a small drawing.

This drawing was James's unique signature. He ended most
of his notes and letters with it: a cartoon of his face, a fringe of
balding hair at the top, a few vertical dashes for his short beard,
cheery round glasses over dots of eyes, and a curve of his irresist-
ible smile. With a few strokes, it captured not only James's like-
ness but also his exuberance. Anyone who knew him recognized
this signature immediately.

Then James told me to write my name on a piece of paper.
The goldsmith could reduce my scribble in size and reproduce it.
So on the oval of James's ring is one word: Susan.

Our rings almost never left our hands—except once, when
James's slipped off his finger into our garbage disposal while
the motor was running. The motor became very noisy. A jeweler

conjured the rescued ring back into shape, with my name scratched but legible, though the ring remained somewhat battered. I told James that this was the symbolic mark of a long and lively marriage.

In his last year of Parkinson's, James lost a great deal of weight. His ring began to slide around on his finger and irritate his thin skin. One day he asked me to remove it and put it in a safe place. (I stashed it in a tiny plastic food storage container on top of my desk.) Occasionally, especially as James's mind began to wander, he would inquire worriedly where his ring was. I would run upstairs to my desk and bring it down to his room. Then he would nod, satisfied he hadn't lost it.

After James died, I did not know what I should do with it. In an earlier era, I might have buried it on his hand. But James was cremated. It was not an heirloom, like a grandmother's diamond engagement ring, that I could pass on to my daughter. Nor did I plan to wear it (as some widows might) on a chain around my neck. I didn't need a reminder of James's commitment. Besides, I had my own ring, with his face, almost burnished into erasure by now, but still there.

James died very early on a Wednesday morning; his funeral was the following Monday; Tuesday our family gathered at the gravesite to deposit his ashes. Between Wednesday and Tuesday, I just knew. I wanted to bury James's wedding ring with his ashes.

On Monday night, after the funeral, I made sure I took the little storage dish, ring inside, and put it on the dining table, ready for the next morning. Early on Tuesday, I drove my daughter, Jenny, on a familiar route toward Lakewood Cemetery. The cemetery, a wooded, rolling piece of land adjacent to the city's most beautiful lake, is less than ten minutes from our house. Although Jenny offered to drive, I wanted to guide the car myself. I felt I was on a precarious and delicate mission I needed to carry out personally.

I wasn't sure exactly what would happen or who would be in charge, but I knew the funeral home had taken James's ashes to Lakewood the previous day. Jenny and I arrived early. Two of James's six children were just getting out of their cars. I instantly identified Lakewood's representative, who I had been told would be waiting on the front steps of the main building. He looked as I expected, wearing a tasteful dark suit, glossily shined shoes, and a solemn expression.

I walked over to greet him. Then I was struck by an awful image. "Oh, my God," I said to Jenny, "I left James's ring on the dining table!" It took me only a few seconds to try to dampen my panic and add, "You stay here. Tell everyone to wait." I got back into the car so I could speed back to our house. Unfortunately—even then I could sense the black humor of this—I immediately found myself trapped behind a patrol car. His car and mine crept in tandem around Lake Harriet. The trip was interminable.

Running fast up our steps, I burst into the house, where my sister and niece were staying. We three had decided to limit the circle at the grave to just James's children and my daughter. In seconds I was at the dining table. The ring was not there. "Kate!" I screamed. "Kate!" My sweet niece is one of the calmest and most competent people I know. Earlier that morning I had told her my plan and shown her James's ring. But what had I done with it then? Where was it? How could I find it? I had to be back at the cemetery right away. Everyone was waiting for me. The ring! How could I bury James without his ring?

"I'll find it," Kate said, and she disappeared upstairs. I had lost all ability to think. In moments she returned with the ring in its container. "On your closet shelf," she said, handing it to me. I ran back down the steps, and this time I *did* speed.

Everyone was standing around at the entrance to the cemetery. I quickly walked over to the Lakewood director. "I want to put this ring in with James's ashes," I said. He nodded and pointed to a black car. "Go ahead," he said. "On the back seat."

Looking back, I'm glad I could not think too clearly about what I was doing. In the car I saw a plain cardboard box. I opened its lid. Inside was a clear plastic Baggie, secured with a tie. The

Baggie looked surprisingly homey, as if it had been pulled out of a kitchen drawer. Through the plastic I could see crumbly gray ashes, looking rather like coarsely ground meal.

I undid the tie. Within the first Baggie was another. A second tie. Then a third Baggie and a third tie. Aware of how unreal this all seemed, I wondered giddily: Such precautions! Would anyone have noticed if a loose ash had escaped? Three Baggies! *Baggies!*

Opening the last Baggie, I grabbed the ring, plunged my hand into the dry, feathery ashes, and buried the ring among them. Carefully I secured each of the three ties and replaced the lid on the cardboard box.

Extricating myself from the back seat, I said, "Okay, I'm ready. Jenny and I will meet you at the grave. I'd like to walk." I couldn't bear to get in a car. I needed fresh air. As I grabbed my daughter's hand, Jenny turned and added reassuringly to everyone, "Don't worry. Mom's a fast walker." She and I strode quickly along the shaded, winding roads, down to the shore of a small lake. I could see ahead of us a little tent covering the gravesite.

When we were all gathered at the excavated space—lined, just large enough, with an urn suspended across it—the Lakewood director showed me how I should empty the Baggie into the urn. Then he tactfully withdrew, standing a short distance away, while the Stagebergs and Toths encircled the grave. We spoke, wept, and did not stay too long.

Five months later in December, I fled the oncoming Minnesota winter for a rental in La Jolla, California. Still dazed from James's death, I felt that I had emerged into a fantasy land—palms, bougainvillea, blue water, sandy beaches, seals, sun-tanned young bodies. I was glad to be there, but I was also often disoriented. I wasn't always sure where I was. I didn't quite know who I was now. I felt lost.

But when I needed to touch ground, I only had to think of a frozen, snow-covered bit of earth in Lakewood Cemetery. Deep below, oblivious to the weather, a gold wedding ring was glowing in the midst of ashes.

CODA

During my years of caregiving, friends sometimes worried about my ability to care for James at home, and sometimes I worried about it myself. Would I be able to keep this commitment? Recently, cleaning out my files, I found the handwritten index card with my vows to James on our wedding day. When I reread that little card, I had my answer. Like all caregivers, I did the best I could.

James, I promise to love and cherish you—to comfort and encourage you—to do what I can about your pain—and to celebrate your joy.

I promise to abide with you in sickness and in health—to live in harmony with you as much as possible—and with the aid of the Higher Power, to support and help you in your deep and admirable desire to live a meaningful life.

I also promise to keep things interesting, to speak up for myself, to laugh at almost all your jokes. In short, I will do the best I can.

ACKNOWLEDGMENTS

I cannot imagine what my last years with James would have been like without help from so many who cared not only for James but for me, with knowledge, attention, friendship, and affection.

We were blessed with two extraordinary doctors, Dr. Tom Davis and Dr. Martha Nance, and a hospice nurse, Annie Watson, who instantly felt like family.

My wonderful aides, some of whom came for a short time and others who saw us through to the end, included Marie Ekstrom, who was there from the very beginning, steadfast and loving, and Eileen Daly, Mary Anne Dols, Sandy Finn, Tiffany Jennings, Kelly Kallstrom, Lori Needels, Anne O'Keefe, Alexandra Roehrdanz, Julie Selmo, and Darlene Zachow.

I owe special thanks to James's son, Frank Stageberg, who gave up many weekend nights so I could sleep and kept me from being stranded more times than I can remember. James's six children, Frank, Beth, Lucy, Jane, Sally, and Anne, and his stepdaughter, Jenny Toth, made sure James knew he was loved.

With inventiveness, craftsmanship, and an artist's eye, Blair Meyers stopped the leaks, righted the helm, and kept our home afloat.

I formed a special bond with women who had once walked this path themselves: Vickie Abrahamson, Barbara Farley, Barbara

Schoening, Anne Simpson, and Felicity Thoet. They continue to cheer me on.

Thank you, Susan King, for listening and especially for assuring me I would one day write again. As always, Julia Friedman Gaff was right there on the end of the long-distance phone line when I needed her. Grateful thanks to the other distant friends who added critical support with their phone calls and e-mail messages.

Helen Gilbert, a gifted therapist, was a lifeline through all the years of James's illness.

Friends who brought me soup, casseroles, roast chicken, and more: you know who you are, and thank you. I will never laugh again at a joke about Minnesota casseroles.

SUSAN ALLEN TOTH is the author of *Blooming: A Small-Town Girlhood, Ivy Days,* and *Leaning into the Wind: A Memoir of Midwest Weather* (Minnesota, 2003), as well as a trilogy on travel in the United Kingdom: *My Love Affair with England, England As You Like It,* and *England for All Seasons.* She has written personal essays and travel pieces for many newspapers and magazines, including the *New York Times, Washington Post,* and *Los Angeles Times.*